AFFORDABLE MEDICARE FOR ALL

American Health Care Is the Problem and
Medicare for All Americans Is the Solution

BARRY G. HOERIG, RN, CCM

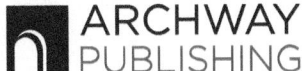
ARCHWAY
PUBLISHING

Archway Publishing books may be ordered through booksellers or by contacting:

Archway Publishing
1663 Liberty Drive
Bloomington, IN 47403
www.archwaypublishing.com
844-669-3957

ISBN: 978-1-6657-0255-3 (sc)
ISBN: 978-1-6657-0256-0 (e)

Library of Congress Control Number: 2021902168

Print information available on the last page.

Archway Publishing rev. date: 04/30/2021

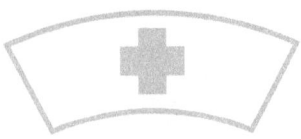

I dedicate this book to all my fellow nurses diligently working every day while improving the lives of their patients.

CONTENTS

I   Introduction 1

II   Capitalism and Healthcare...................................... 16

III   Medicare For All: X=Y 33

IV   Medicare For All and Taxes 38

V   Medicare For All and Private Insurance 63

VI   Medicare For All and The Veterans Administration 69

VII   Medicare For All and Corrections............................ 81

VIII Medicare For All and Politics.................................. 84

IX   Modern American Slavery 95

X   House Bill 1384.. 100

XI   Implementing Medicare For All............................. 105

XII   Take Aways and Next Steps 109

References 113

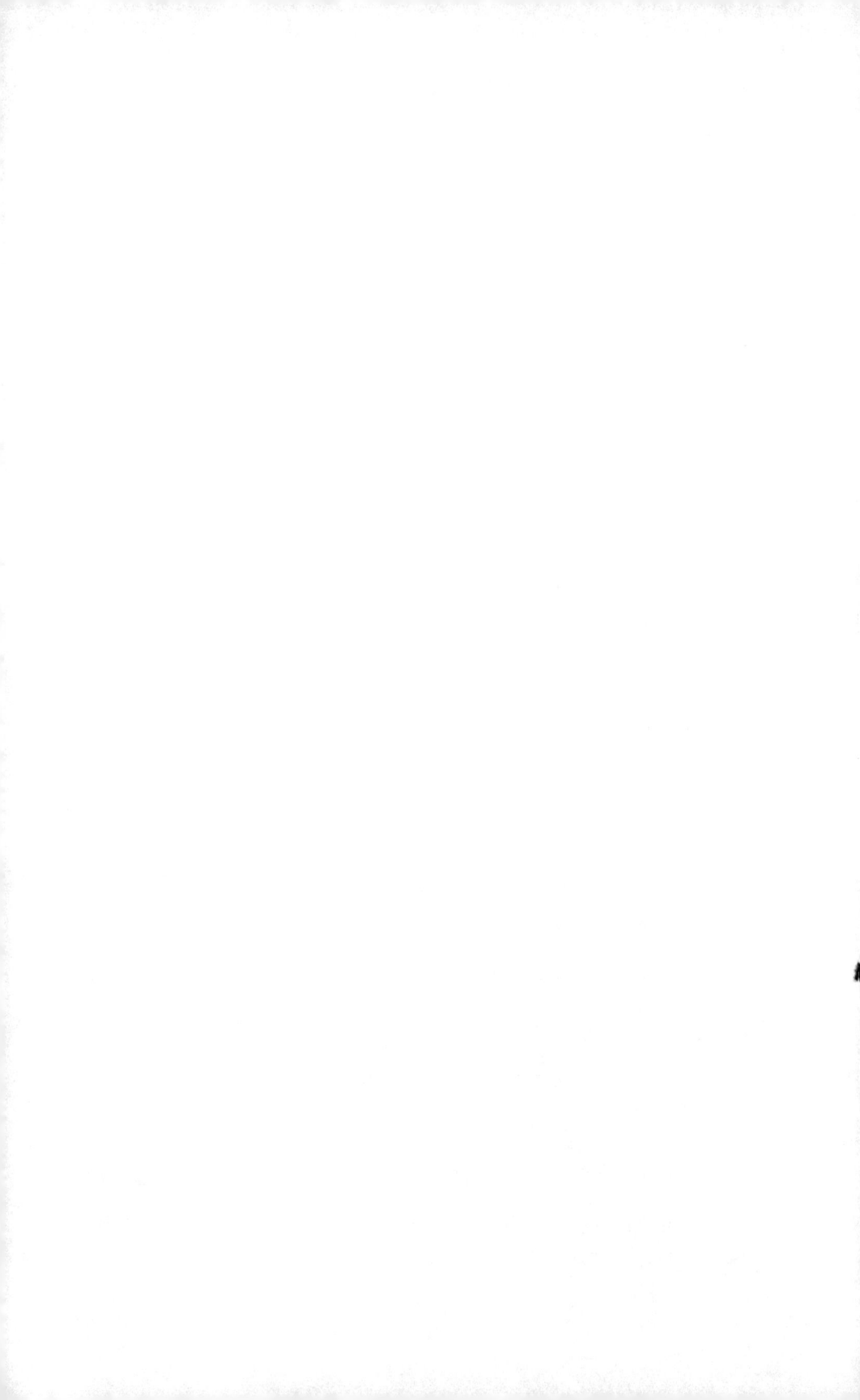

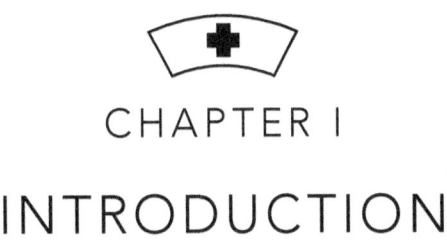

CHAPTER 1

INTRODUCTION

Newspapers, television news programs, and news websites fill airwaves and content regarding the excessive expense of American health care and the proposal to transition to "Medicare For All" (M4A). Many internet posts attempt to respond to the question, "How are you going to pay for that?" This book answers that question with mathematical calculations and proposals without political hyperbole.

Let us first reframe and restate the question, "How are you going to pay for that?" to "How will Americans pay for equal health-care access for all Americans?" Revising the question clarifies some realities. *You* now become *us*, focusing the question on how we Americans share responsibility for ourselves as a nation. We claim the value of everyone being created equal, so I propose taking a huge step toward actual equality. Medicare For All results in all Americans benefiting from the exact same basic health insurance coverage regardless of age, race, gender, religion, residence, birth, sexual orientation, disability, or whatever.

Another clarification is the expectation that all American adults contribute financially to the coverage. No freeloaders. No exceptions. That includes all corporations, governments, and employers of any sort. I will examine how one of the great economic inequalities of American capitalism exists because polluting industries receive indirect subsidies by not contributing tax revenues toward health care in proportion to the healthcare risks they create. Producers of coal, oil, and other toxins avoid paying additional taxes while producing toxic products and reap subsidies via various tax breaks awarded by politicians. Those industries will argue that increasing their taxes will spell certain doom for us all, when the probability exists that they can manage paying additional taxes by reducing spending on stock buybacks, stock dividends, exorbitant executive compensation, and political party and political candidate donations.

As I already promised, this book calculates the cost of every American and legal resident within the United States of America receiving Medicare coverage at the current coverage level. I anticipate many political responses to my arguments. I am extremely interested in input from my fellow Americans regarding refining the proposed mathematics. I am not interested in political comments lacking support from verifiable mathematical data. Those sharing data and facts correcting my formulas have my ear. Otherwise, please share unsupported political commentary with those interested in hearing unsupported political opinion.

WHO IS "ALL"?

Medicare For All means health insurance coverage for all American citizens and legal residents of the United States. M4A would result in members of the United States Congress, the President of the United States, and all members of the Supreme Court having the same basic health insurance coverage as the lowliest impoverished homeless Americans. Wealthy Americans living in spacious mansions would enjoy the same coverage level as the servants maintaining their households. Puerto Ricans would have the same coverage as Alaskans. The residents of the Gold Coast of Chicago would have the same coverage as the residents of South Chicago. The one group that would enjoy better benefits than other Americans would be veterans and active-duty military service members, which I explain further in a separate chapter.

"All" includes all American citizens, legal residents of the USA, and all persons residing within all United States territories. The USA includes all fifty states, all American territories, and every American military base throughout the world. Every American would receive coverage, and therefore every American would contribute.

"All" includes all current health-care insurance plans. Some M4A proponents demand completely eliminating private health insurance. I argue that doing so is both politically and practically undesirable and unattainable. Private health insurance plans provide essential services to beneficiaries and government. Eliminating private insurance plans would both make M4A implementation unnecessarily tedious and onerous and would greatly delay implementation of the transition to M4A.

"All" includes coverage of all incarcerated American citizens and incarcerated legal aliens. I will discuss how coverage of the incarcerated will greatly benefit the nation in a separate chapter.

WHAT MEDICARE FOR ALL IS NOT

One of the requirements for mathematical equations is that values and relationships are standardized and stable. The specification of "Who is all?" can be regarded as inclusionary criteria. Now we will discuss exclusionary criteria, or clarifications regarding what is not included in these M4A calculations.

M4A does not include any changes in current Medicare coverage. That means the current level of coverage for Medicare Part A, Part B, Part D, and Medicare Advantage plans remains unchanged. For those not already aware of the different parts of Medicare coverage, here is a summary:

- Part A covers hospitalization with a standardized out-of-pocket cost; home health, and hospice care; inpatient skilled nursing; and inpatient rehab services.
- Part B covers 80 percent of outpatient services such as physician office visits, lab tests, X-rays, and other diagnostic testing, after payment of an annual deductible.
- Part D covers prescription drugs with varied copays depending on the cost of the drug. Part D has a deductible that must be met at the beginning of each year. Persons with high medication

costs eventually hit a "donut hole" where they lose coverage and pay 100 percent for medications; after they have spent so much on medications, they reach the other side of the "donut hole," and prescription drug coverage resumes with lowered copays.

- Medicare Advantage plans are HMOs and other similar combination plans where Medicare pays a monthly premium to the plan. Part A and Part B coverages are combined into one plan, and Part D prescription coverage may also be included.

M4A does not involve any reduction of benefits to veterans or active military.

M4A does not involve the provision of coverage outside the borders of the USA, as overseas military bases are considered within the borders of the USA.

M4A does not include coverage of persons illegally present within the USA.

M4A does not cover legally visiting foreigners to the USA.

M4A does not include coverage of elective abortions for non-life-threatening situations. It also does not include any in vitro fertilization, artificial insemination, or other artificial means of human reproduction.

M4A excludes health insurance coverage while traveling outside the borders of the USA. For example, if one travels from New York City to an American military base in Germany, while in transit between those locations, there is no Medicare coverage. However, upon arrival at the military base in Germany, Medicare coverage resumes if the medical service is provided on-base.

M4A does not mean "one-payer" health insurance coverage. Medicare Part A has an out-of-pocket cost for hospitalizations, Medicare Part B already provides 80/20 coverage, and Part D already requires prescription copays. So, at a minimum, there will be two payers: Medicare and the beneficiary. I envision that most Americans under M4A would be covered by three payers: Medicare first, then a private insurance plan, and then the beneficiary, who would pay any remaining out-of-pocket costs.

M4A does not mean allowing excessive compensation for services or products. The taxpayer should not pay for multimillion-dollar compensation of corporate executives or pay excessive prescription drug costs. Drug manufacturers may pay their executives whatever compensation their governing boards determine; however, the manufacturer must not charge the American taxpayer excessive rates to reward excessive executive compensation.

"SINGLE-PAYER" IS POLITICAL DOUBLESPEAK

In May 2019, the Congressional Budget Office (CBO) of the US Congress published a report, *Key Design Components and Considerations for Establishing a Single-Payer Health Care System*. On page 1 of the report, the CBO defines these four characteristics of a "single-payer" health-care system:

1. The government is responsible for operations of the plan.
2. Persons covered by the health plan are required to contribute to financing of the plan.
3. Funding and costs are a portion of the government's budget.
4. Private insurance plays a small role and supplements the coverage provided by the government.

If you have been keeping count, you have already noticed that the CBO's description of a "single-payer" plan includes three payers, not one. Those three payers are the government, the people covered by the plan, and private insurers. If there is any "single payer" for health care, it is the taxpayer paying the taxes directly from their paychecks or paying the taxes on goods and services purchased. Therefore, let us dispense with the nonsense and doublespeak of "single-payer." There is no single-payer, and Medicare For All will include all these payers:

A. The federal government via the Centers for Medicare and Medicaid Services, the Social Security Administration, and the Internal Revenue Service.

B. Employees via payroll deduction, taxable products and services, and deductibles, copays, and coinsurance out-of-pocket costs.

C. Employers via matching payroll taxes, taxable goods and services, and payment for health insurance plans that supplement basic Medicare coverage.

D. Private insurance plans covering health-care services and products not covered by the primary plan and covering visitors to the USA ineligible for coverage by the national plan.

On page 4 of the report, six nations with "single-payer" health-care systems are listed: Australia, Canada, Denmark, England, Sweden, and Taiwan. For Canada, the health insurance plan is administered not by the Canadian federal government, but by each province or territory, which means there are thirteen different payers, as each province or territory is a payer. In addition, each province has differences with coverage and eligibility, and some have waiting periods before a new resident can enroll with the provincial or territorial plan. In addition, when Canadians travel outside their province of residency to another Canadian province or territory, their province of residency is billed for health-care services received in other provinces, and their province will only pay the bill if that service is also covered by the province of residency. For residents of Quebec, the provincial health insurance plan has agreements with some foreign nations that allow Quebec residents to use their Quebec health insurance coverage while temporarily working in that other nation. So, even though Canada has "universal" health-care coverage in that all Canadian citizens are covered by a government-managed health insurance plan, there are numerous actual payers.

Therefore, I am proposing universal coverage for all American citizens and legal residents, not a single-payer system. No one else is truly proposing a "single payer" system either.

POSITIVE IMPACTS

The formula excludes the financial impact of savings realized from improved quality and efficiency from eliminating current coverage overlaps and coverage gaps. I am unable to include those estimations of the financial impacts of such improvements as that information is not readily available. I list those impacts here and will explain the improvements from each in subsequent chapters. I anticipate all these improvements:

- Improved access to primary care services for all Americans.
- Improved access to healthcare for veterans, especially for veterans that live in rural areas, or other areas requiring significant travel to reach a VA healthcare center.
- Reduction of federal and state administration costs for Medicaid-eligible persons.
- Reduced billing and claims costs for providers and health insurance plans.
- Improved and consistent revenue streams to providers allowing providers to better serve currently underserved persons and areas.
- Reduction of administrative costs for Medicare, providers, employers, and health insurance plans.
- Better data collection of illness and death, known as morbidity and mortality, allowing the Centers for Disease Control to track and predict illness and infection more accurately and reliably.
- Long-term financial stability and reliability of Medicare funding.
- Reduced health insurance premiums paid by both individuals and employers.
- Reduced workers compensation premiums for employers.
- Reduced legal liability and reduced liability insurance premiums for physicians and all healthcare providers.
- Reduced automobile and motor vehicle insurance premiums.
- Improved financial viability of all healthcare providers, especially for those serving economically disadvantaged areas.

MATH AND ECONOMICS

I will describe the mathematical and economic changes needed for enacting and implementing a workable Medicare For All law. My focus explains how a properly shared tax structure across American commercial activity results in sufficiently funding Medicare For All at the current level of Medicare coverage. The basis for each calculation and tax proposal has been retrieved from readily available websites, so that anyone with internet access may verify the data and calculations.

Let us now review the economic systems of current and past human history, known as economisms. The economisms are:

FEUDALISM

A "lord" or other master owns and controls the land, and landholders are organized into a hierarchal aristocracy resulting in monarchs and other "royalty" and various lesser titled persons and families. The primary means of production is non-mechanized agriculture and most of the populace, called serfs or peasants, are indentured to the master. The master provides protection from attack via castles and forts and the profits from the sale and trade of agricultural products returns to the master. Although oil production is the commercial activity controlled by royalty, instead of agriculture, Saudi Arabia is a best current example of a persisting feudalistic society. The Saudi royal family controls the economic activity of the entire nation, and all non-royals are obligated to be productive for the sake of the royal family. The Saudi Royal Family calls the shots while the Saudi citizens live with the consequences.

SOCIALISM

Partially free markets may exist, but the government tightly controls primary commercial activity and directly owns and operates large commercial corporations. The members of government may be "elected," however, government also strictly controls candidacy for government offices so that the persons elected already support the economic and social dogma of the government. Socialistic nations encounter a great deal of difficulty managing severe external threats because the rigidity of thought and action suppresses the innovation needed for adaptation to a changing world. Nazism is the extreme example of socialism both in its operation and defeat. The Nazis could be successful while being the aggressor and conquering their neighbors and harvesting the resources of the conquered. However, once more determined, and superior opponents counter attacked, they exhausted their resources and could not develop the creativity of changing tactics and adapting.

COMMUNISM

Communist governments control and manage all aspects of commercial and economic activity. Essentially, all citizens of a communist nation are government employees. Although Karl Marx and Friedrich Engels attempted to address the social and economic disparities of crony capitalism and the Gilded Age, their beliefs and theories possessed a major flaw. They failed accounting for the natural human tendency and need of positive reward for work and effort. Communism eliminates rewarding the individual based on personal productivity and expects individual productivity for the state regardless of level of compensation. Communism also shares a common defect with crony capitalism in how money and resources become concentrated and controlled by the few elite and highly placed government officials while the masses subsist on minimal compensation. Eventually, so many people lose their motivation for productivity that eventually the economic activity of the nation collapses because there are simply insufficient workers willing to work at a satisfactorily productive level to maintain the economy, and a severe economic depression accompanies the collapse of the government. The Soviets were unwilling to modify their nation to allow it to survive. In contrast, The People's Republic of China integrated some capitalistic principles which allowed economic growth and lifted hundreds of millions of Chinese citizens out of poverty.

STATISM

Also known as Nazism and fascism, concentrates all power with the state and eliminates personal freedoms. Statism could be described as socialism on steroids. There is no pretense of personal rights or liberties.

And Statism is like Feudalism in that a select elite control and manage the entire national economy and government. Elections are shams as the entrenched governing elite select and limit the candidates, and a candidate will be selected only if they already support the dogma of the established elite.

WELFARE STATE

The welfare state assures the economic success and stability of all citizens. There are open elections and personal freedoms including property rights. Welfare states mimic capitalistic nations as the right to own and accumulate property and wealth are allowed but are more difficult to achieve due to the high taxes. High taxation supports the numerous social support programs operated by the government and are essential for maintenance of a welfare state. Welfare states reduce poverty by utilizing high taxes on the wealthy to provide guaranteed incomes and benefits for the lower classes. Welfare states enjoy economic and social stability but tend to stifle innovation.

CAPITALISM

Capitalism, although the strongest of the economisms, possesses a dark side. Free markets are the hallmark of capitalism, with individuals permitted to accumulate as much money and property as desired and possible. The major strength of capitalism is the strong rewards and incentives for productivity and innovation. Consistently throughout American history, hard workers creating new services and products thrive. The major weakness of capitalism is the promotion of worsening income equality as elites and wealthy gain ever more wealth while the lower classes struggle to meet daily financial obligations because their lower incomes are consumed by progressively increasing living expenses. The Federal Reserve Bank exemplifies this process of classist and racist inequality. By keeping interest rates exceeding low, low-interest loans fuel expanding real estate purchasing and speculation, augmenting escalating real estate prices and rents. As housing costs increase at a rate greater than the rate of wage increases, the lower classes spend a greater percentage of their incomes on housing, while the wealthy enjoy the benefits of greater sale values of their properties.

Another strength of capitalism is how integration of an innovation into the economy usually results in an eventual reduction of cost, eventually allowing all classes of citizens affordability of that product or service. For example, when the automobile was first introduced in the 19th century, only the wealthy could afford one, the same way mostly the wealthy can afford to purchase a Tesla automobile today. However, Henry Ford revolutionized industrialization and the automobile industry by refining manufacturing and reducing the cost of production significantly, thereby reducing the purchase price of a Ford automobile. Once the purchase price of a car came within the means of most Americans, Ford's production and success expanded dramatically, eventually replacing the horse and carriage as the primary means of transportation. Ford also began paying a significantly improved wage to his employees, which better allowed his employees to become purchasers of Ford automobiles. Note how the purchase price of fully electric vehicles has been decreasing, allowing more people to become purchasers. Such is the great strength and power of capitalism.

The great sin of capitalism is worsening income inequality between social classes. As the wealthy become wealthier, their greater accumulation comes at the expense of the middle and lower classes. Left unchecked, eventually the economy collapses into recessions and depressions because the middle and lower classes have fewer funds to pay for living expenses as those expenses escalate while their incomes either decrease or stagnate. Such is what happened with the Great Depression of 1929 and the Great Recession of 2009. The wealthy become wealthier by decreasing financial resources to the lower classes. In 2009, a major mechanism was corporations eliminating pension plans and reducing healthcare coverage to improve their bottom lines and therefore their stock performance. The company elites, who own much of the company stock, become enriched by reducing their employment expenses with lower healthcare and pension costs, which are shifted to employees. Healthcare cost increases cancel out wage gains. The elite classes effectively transfer money and wealth from the other social classes to themselves. Then, the wealthy use their additional wealth to continue to drive the stock markets up, until eventually the speculative bubble bursts and the stock market dramatically declines, endangering the financial health of everyone. Federal tax policy encourages the cycle of boom and bust by lowering tax percentage on the wealthy, providing more funds for speculative stock purchases and buy backs. While the economy booms, everything is wine and roses. But, when the economy tanks, the middle and lower classes endure greater financial suffering.

The same pattern and process continues today. General Motors closes factories and lays off workers, whose federal income taxes bailed out General Motors, preventing its complete dissolution only 10 years ago. Medicare For All balances the distribution of wealth among the social classes by reducing the financial burden of expensive American healthcare on those who have the least means of affording it. As a bonus, I will mathematically demonstrate how the additional taxes for Medicare for All will result in an overall reduction of labor expenses for businesses.

Let me repeat that: As a bonus, I will mathematically demonstrate how the additional taxes for Medicare for All will result in an overall reduction of labor expenses for businesses.

MY PHILOSOPHY

Now that "single-payer" and the various socioeconomic types have been reviewed, I now proffer an explanation of my personal philosophy, explaining so that all readers understand my perspective and motives.

Simply, my philosophy is lacking in any intent to influence you, or anyone, in any coercive or deceptive manner. I offer facts and figures supported by calculations and retrievable references. I am hopeful that every American will appreciate and understand how a properly structured and funded Medicare For All benefits all Americans. Yes, I do want to persuade you to favor my offered version of Medicare For All, but I want your favor not because I act as an authority, but rather because you genuinely agree that despite the financial adjustments and tax increases required to properly fund Medicare For All, you agree that Medicare for All benefits yourself, your family, your community, your state and your country.

ABBREVIATIONS

Throughout this book, I use abbreviations extensively, because the world of healthcare and healthcare finance overflows with abbreviations and acronyms. Here is a listing of the abbreviations and acronyms used:

CBO = Congressional Budget Office

CDC = Centers for Disease Control and Prevention

CMS = Centers for Medicare and Medicaid Services

EA = Ethyl alcohol for human consumption

EN = Hydrocarbons burned in internal combustion engines

ER = Emergency Room or Emergency Department

FDIC = Federal Deposit Insurance Corporation

FF = Fossil Fuels/hydrocarbons burned in furnaces

FICA = Federal Insurance Contribution Act

GDP = Gross Domestic Product

GOV = Other government healthcare programs

HC = Hydrocarbon related

HFCS = High Fructose Corn Syrup

HHS = US Dept of Health and Human Services

HI = Health insurance

HMO = Health Maintenance Organization

IT = Income Tax (in addition to payroll taxes)

LLC = Limited Liability Corporation

M4A = Medicare For All

MA = Medicare Advantage plans

MC = Medicare

MD = Medicaid programs

Na = Salt/Foods with added sodium chloride

NHE = National Health Expenditure

NHR = National Health Revenue

Ni = Nicotine/Nicotine-containing products

OP = Out of pocket expenses

OTC = Over the counter (nonprescription) medication

P4P = Pay for Performance

PI = Private health insurance

POW = Prisoner of War

PPO = Preferred Provider Organization

PR = Health insurance premiums

PX = Payroll taxes

PXe = Payroll taxes paid by employers

PXw = Payroll taxes paid by workers

RAC = Recovery Audit Contractor

RN = Registered Nurse

SE = Stock Exchanges

SUV = Sport utility vehicles (includes crossover)

Su = Sugars

Tn = Toxin

TR = TriCare for Life health insurance plan

UCLA = University of California Los Angeles

UM = Utilization Management

URL = Uniform Resource Locator

USA = United State of America and territories

USSR = Union of Soviet Socialist Republics

VA = The Veterans Administration

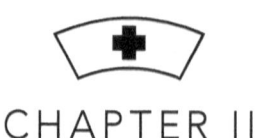

CHAPTER II

CAPITALISM AND HEALTHCARE

AMERICAN HEALTHCARE IS NOT CAPITALISM

In their book, *The Case Against Socialism*, Senator Rand Paul and Kelly Ashley Paul nicely describe and warn against the dangers of socialism. They specifically cite on the book jacket, "free spending policies like Medicare for All," while not applying the recognized hazards of capitalism and failing to recognize how the current system of prescription healthcare in America is not capitalistic. I especially enjoyed the comment on the back of the book jacket by Judge Andrew Napolitano: "No U.S. senator in the modern era can rival Senator Rand Paul's fidelity to the first principles of the free market." Let us compare "free market capitalism" and the actual world of American-style healthcare. However, the Rands acknowledge how the current American economy blends capitalism and socialism.

THERE IS NO "FREE MARKET"
FOR MOST HEALTHCARE.

In actual free markets, the consumer freely chooses providers, products and services based on factors such as convenience, preferences, price, and quality. For example, in my neighborhood, my two primary shopping destinations are Walmart and Safeway. I buy sundries and household products at Walmart because there is no significant quality difference between the two stores, with better prices for those items at Walmart, and with minimal driving transportation cost. But I buy groceries, especially produce, at Safeway because of the significantly better selection and quality of fresh foods at Safeway. I willingly pay more at Safeway for the foods I enjoy so that I get the quality I desire. Such is true free market capitalism. I choose where I shop, the items I purchase, and I factor in price comparisons as part of the decision-making process. I am not burdened with a requirement to shop or purchase at either store. I go to any store stocking the items I desire, and I price compare between available vendors. And Safeway sweetens their pie by rewarding my purchases with gas discounts at their gas station when I fuel my car. The Pauls mention the importance of pricing as a means of feedback for both producers and consumers in a free market capitalistic economy. I suspect there is no more important criteria of true capitalism than transparent pricing, as at both stores, the price of each item, including a pricing ratio (per ounce, per pound, etc.) is displayed on the shelf or display case.

Another prime characteristic of capitalism links quality and price. Using automobiles as an example, a Mercedes Benz fetches a higher price than a Chevy because the perceived better quality of the Mercedes by consumers. The automobile buyer expects the higher price of the Mercedes Benz because of both the market reputation and the engineering and manufacturing differences of one compared to the other.

Social class affects purchasing decisions. Upper class persons, with greater income and financial assets, trend towards purchasing the Mercedes Benz because they possess the money to afford the purchase, and as a member of a higher social class, they have an expectation from the supplier to provide a higher quality product. So, supply and demand have several different relationships to each other. Higher class consumers pay more for a higher quality product or service, while lower class consumers pay for and expect a lesser quality product or service. The higher quality satisfies the demand by higher class consumers while the demand by lower class consumers is satisfied by the lesser priced and lesser quality product or service. Consumers feel cheated if the quality of the product is unusually less than the price paid, based upon their expectation as a member of whichever social group they belong. The wealthy, when they purchase the Mercedes, expect the quality of a Mercedes, and feel cheated if the vehicle delivered does not meet that expectation. Likewise, the quality of a Chevy satisfies the expectation of the middle-class consumer purchasing a Chevy.

For most American healthcare, a reverse relationship between quality and price exists. Lower class healthcare consumers, such as the poor, homeless and working poor, pay a higher price for healthcare services because they are either not insured, or are underinsured. Especially the uninsured, billed full charges for medical care, are expected to pay more for less because they lack the luxury of getting discounted rates from a health insurance plan. The poor and uninsured also suffer from lower healthcare quality from the limitations of access to basic services such as a primary care physician and prescription medicines. When an uninsured American goes to the pharmacy to fill a prescription, often they pay more for the same drug than the customer next in line, when that next customer has coverage by a health insurance plan that pays for a prescription at a discounted rate. The same person who must pay a higher price because of their lack of health insurance does not have that problem when purchasing an automobile. The lower classes may purchase vehicles with some reasonable consumer choice because there are plenty of automobile dealers with plenty of vehicles that are priced affordably for them. For the healthcare uninsured, the exact opposite is true. They endure a lesser availability of providers, and then must pay more for either the same or a lesser quality medication or healthcare service. It's the reverse of capitalism. Hence, American prescription healthcare is anticapitalistic.

Over the counter (OTC) medications are a good example of how healthcare can be very capitalist in an incredibly positive way. I suffer from chronic back pain. I despise narcotics and other prescription medications like muscle relaxers which cause too many side effects that interfere with my ability to work. So, for many years, I managed by chronic pain with OTC medications such as acetaminophen and naproxen. But both medications have limitations as to how much pain relief I experience. When lidocaine 5% prescription pain patches became available, I was excited because I thought I may have found a medication that would provide better pain relief than the acetaminophen and naproxen.

My hopes were dashed when I learned that even with the health insurance coverage from my employer, I would pay about $400 per month for a full month supply of the pain patches, which I simply cannot afford. Note how the monthly price for a non-narcotic pain medication approximately equals a monthly car loan payment, even with health insurance coverage. Even though the 5% lidocaine pain relief patch has been on the market for several years, I have not seen a price reduction and the price of the prescription-strength patches remains outside my affordability.

Then, about one and a half years ago, nonprescription strength 4% lidocaine patches became available as an OTC medication throughout America. What a game changer for me! Even though not full prescription strength, the OTC strength lidocaine provides sufficiently improved pain relief. When the OTC patches first became available in the pharmacy, the cost for a month's supply, even though not covered by health insurance, was about $150 per month, which now made the option within my price range. For less than half of the out-of-pocket cost of the prescription strength patches, I get a product that provides the pain relief I need.

It gets even better as a shining example of capitalism at work. There are several manufacturers of the OTC lidocaine patches, so every few months, I would again price compare, then switch to purchasing the OTC lidocaine patch with a lesser per-patch price. Originally, I was paying approximate $2.50 per patch. Recently, another manufacturer of the OTC patches began supplying patches online, at a lower cost than what I was able to obtain in a pharmacy. Online, my per-patch price is now approximately $1. Note that the price reduction for the OTC patches, in approximately a year and a half, has reduced in price by 60%.

Isn't capitalism wonderful? Nonprescription healthcare is capitalistic, whereas prescription healthcare is very much anticapitalistic.

So, let us pretend we truly experience a free market for prescription healthcare in America, and I need to obtain a refill of a prescription for a cholesterol-lowering medication. In a true free market, I would compare prices between the available pharmacies in my area, then choose which pharmacy had the better price, and purchase the refill at that pharmacy. I do not currently enjoy such freedom though.

I enjoy freedom of choice only if I do not have health insurance and pay cash for the refill. But, without health insurance, I pay the highest prices because various state and federal laws and regulations require that healthcare products and services be charged at a consistent rate, with discounts provided to those with health insurance coverage. The same applies to hospitals and physicians. They charge inflated standard rates, discounted under contracts with the insurance plans, but not discounted for the uninsured who must self-pay. Please note how this arrangement is the exact opposite of a true free market. In free markets, providers and products compete for consumer attention and purchasing, which tends to promote price reductions, not price increases. Pricing transparency, essential indicators of free markets, remains mostly absent from the American version of prescription healthcare.

I lack true freedom of choice regarding where I obtain a prescription refill because of my employer's health insurance coverage. My employer permits only two options—enroll in the HMO (health maintenance organization) with no deduction from my paycheck or enroll in a PPO (preferred provider organization) for a monthly deduction of about $400 from my paycheck.

The PPO allows the choice of any provider I wish, but I pay more both from my paycheck and for each healthcare service to obtain that freedom. Plus, there are no third or fourth health insurance options allowed by my employer. So of course, I chose the HMO because of the lower costs out of my pocket and paycheck. But the HMO restricts which physicians and hospitals I may use and decides the copays and deductibles for me. I lose the ability of price comparison. I no longer enjoy freedom of choice, the linchpin of capitalism, because my employer restricts my choices of health insurance coverage and the insurance plan restricts the pricing and providers. An equivalent scenario would be if my employer restricted which stores their employees may shop for groceries and sundries. Prices would not be posted on the shelves, requiring I make purchasing decisions without knowing the cost before I choose. Then, I learn the price I am responsible for paying when each item as scanned at the checkout counter. And the customer in line before or after me would pay completely different prices for the exact same item.

In the November 4, 2019 issue of *Time* magazine, Grant Burningham describes both capitalistic and non-capitalistic economic systems of American healthcare. Burningham reports about Anthony Di Franco and the team at Counter Culture Labs in Oakland, California working at duplicating modern insulin production at a much lower cost. The positive part of capitalism regards how Counter Culture Labs attempts that goal because the cost of recombinant DNA technology has progressively decreased as more companies are able to provide the lab services needed, and compete against one another, which progressively lowers the price.

Then, Burningham explains how three Big Pharma companies control most of the insulin market and tweak the formulations periodically, maintaining their patents, and therefore the higher prices for those products. Burningham further explains when a patient died because the patient could not afford to pay $1300 per month for treatment of his diabetes and how 13.2% of Americans prescribed insulin do not take it as prescribed, according to the CDC. As a registered nurse, having taken care of innumerable patients with diabetes, I personally attest to the reality that many persons with diabetes do not properly take prescribed insulin and oral medications because they simply cannot afford to do so. For them, it truly is a decision to not take the medicine as prescribed so that they will have enough money to pay rent and buy food.

I also personally attest to Burningham's report and the statistics he cites from the CDC. For many years I worked home health, and I would admit about four or five patients weekly, after their discharge home from either a hospital or rehab facility. Most patients required reporting to their physician that they were either not taking a prescribed medication at all, or not taking it correctly. And the most common reason in my experience that a patient does not take medication correctly is the unaffordability of the medication at the pharmacy. The patient becomes labeled as "noncompliant," and endures negative judgements by healthcare professionals, leading us to physician prescribing practices, the next factor affecting excess medication costs.

Generally, most physicians prescribe medications, devices, and treatments to gain the greatest benefits for their patients. However, I have not ever personally witnessed or heard of any physician asking a patient or their family if they could afford the drug, device or procedure prescribed. And it completely misses the reality that a person's financial health greatly contributes to personal health. If one does not take prescribed insulin because they lack the income to afford it, then die because they did not take the prescribed insulin, financial health profoundly impacts personal health.

Let us examine the anticapitalism of physician prescribing practices. These steps describe the first-time prescription of insulin for many patients:

I.   While hospitalized, an elevated blood sugar is discovered during lab testing.

II.   The physician treating the hospitalized patient, a hospitalist, is a stranger to the patient and the family as most primary care physicians no longer perform hospital rounds.

III. The hospitalist decides which type of insulin shall be prescribed, and the method of injection, which is usually by insulin pen injector, rather than by needle-and-syringe.

IV.   No one discusses with the patient or family medication choices and options, and upon discharge home, the patient is issued a medication list and any new prescriptions are electronically transmitted to their preferred pharmacy. Home health nursing is often ordered teaching of the insulin injection and routine diabetic self-care.

V. The patient or family member arrives at the pharmacy to pick up the filled insulin prescription. Commonly, the prescription cannot be filled because the insulin prescribed is not on the formulary restriction of the prescription drug plan, or the insulin requires prior authorization, which has not yet been done because either the hospitalist did not complete the prior authorization request form, or the pharmacy is waiting for the prescription drug plan to respond to the prior authorization request. Or, if the prior authorization has been approved, the patient still cannot afford the high copay, and if uninsured, cannot afford the full cash price.

VI. The patient, now at home, has no insulin. The home health nurse arrives and cannot teach proper insulin injection.

VII. The nurse notifies the primary care physician of the patient's inability to inject the insulin because of no insulin supply due to either the prior authorization is not complete, or the patient cannot afford the price of the insulin prescribed by the hospitalist.

VIII. The primary care physician must now decide whether to proceed with the prior authorization request or prescribe a different insulin approved by the insurance plan's formulary and hope the patient can afford the insulin. In some cases, the patient never receives the insulin at all because the prior authorization problem becomes intractable, or the patient simply cannot afford the price of any insulin.

A MORE CAPITALISTIC MEDICARE FOR ALL

As the Pauls admit, American economics and society are a blend of capitalism and socialism. The trick is the challenge of blending both in proper proportions which provides the best of both while minimizing the worst of both. Here are some ideas to achieve such as masterful recipe:

1. Once implemented, taxes would cover the cost of the 80% of Medicare-covered services for every American citizen and legal resident. The current Medicare premiums for Part B and Part D coverage would be eliminated. Premiums would exist only for Medicare supplemental coverage, which could be paid by individuals, employers, or state Medicaid programs. Or, in the case of veterans and active military, Tricare provides Medicare supplement coverage.

2. Taxes would cover Tricare coverage for all active military and their families and all veterans as a secondary coverage to Medicare. Hence, active military, their families and veterans enjoy complete Medicare coverage without any premiums paid directly by themselves, an employer, or any state.

3. Employers offer paying for Medicare supplemental coverage for their employees and employee's families. Employers would be allowed either offering a flat-rate benefit towards the premium, or contract with health insurance plans to provide the supplemental benefits. Insurance companies would have the option of either offering a combined Medicare MA plan, like the current arrangement for Medicare Advantage plans, or to offer a straight supplemental insurance.

4. Insurance companies retain marketing directly to consumers and contracting with Medicare to provide combination Medicare Advantage plans. Insurance plans would include premium, copay and other out-of-pocket costs in their advertising and marketing activities. Insurance plans enjoy free reign with devising any combination health insurance plans they wish, providing the minimum Medicare standard coverage continues as it currently does for Medicare MA plans.

5. Congress legislates CMS develop a basic prescription drug coverage accepted at any pharmacy in the USA. Insurance plans and employers could offer enhanced prescription drug coverage benefits to employers and directly to consumers. Prescription drug costs would be negotiated between pharmaceutical

companies and Congress. Insurance plans could negotiate lower prescription drug costs whenever possible.

6. States may alter their current Medicaid programs creating Medicare supplement plans for low income and otherwise Medicaid-eligible residents. Each state could contract with private insurance plans to provide the coverage, and the state would pay premiums to cover each Medicaid-eligible resident. Each state develops its own method of taxation covering the cost of Medicaid supplemental insurance.

7. Physician prescriptions become "shopped." That is, instead of a prescription being directly transmitted to a pharmacy, the patient and family would price compare with available pharmacies the cost of the prescription. The patient and family would make a consumer decision based upon cost and quality comparisons. Shopping prescriptions would also apply to other medical services such as elective surgeries, cancer chemotherapy, home health and hospice and skilled nursing facilities and outpatient services. Physicians discuss costs of care prior to prescribing. Patient consent for taking medications, ancillary services and medical procedures includes revealing the cost of the drug, service, or procedure before the signing of the consent.

8. Insurance companies compete to provide coverage of Medicare and Medicaid benefits and operate and compete across state lines. Congress and the state legislatures would redefine the regulatory relationship between insurance plans and the states to accommodate that competition.

9. Appropriately educated and certified consumer advocates assist patients and families with making healthcare purchasing choices.

10. Congress reviews and modifies the Stark and Anti-Kickback laws allowing more transparent communication of pricing and choices to consumers. Physicians may have a financial interest in healthcare providers to which they refer, but they fully disclose that interest prior to prescription and disclose the price of the prescribed drug or service before the patient and family consent

to the treatment. Drug manufacturers enjoy more freedom with offering discounts and assistance directly to consumers and insurance plans.

11. Price gouging for medical products and services becomes criminalized. The practice of purchasing a drug or device patent solely for the purpose of excessively increasing the price and profits becomes forbidden as the form of price gouging that it is. Companies developing new drugs and medical devices receive a reasonable profit and return on investment but justify their costs of development as part of a negotiation process with Congress setting the price within the USA.

MORE CAPITALISTIC HEALTHCARE DECISION MAKING

Let us now revisit the hospitalized patient prescribed insulin. A more capitalistic medical decision-making process occurs:

I.   The hospitalized patient continues treatment by the hospitalist.
II. When deciding which insulin to prescribe, the hospitalist obtains this information before discussing discharge medications with the patient and family:
  a. All the available types of insulin appropriate for the current medical diagnosis.
  b. The cost of each insulin, including both the total cost and the patient's out-of-pocket cost for each type of insulin.
  c. The requirement for any prior authorization and the process for submitting and obtaining approval of the prior authorization.
III. The hospitalist, with the discharge planner nurse, and possibly a pharmacist, assist the patient and family with reviewing the choices available including the types of insulins, costs, and prior authorization considerations.
IV. The patient and family choose which insulin they can best afford. The hospitalist prescribes the insulin the patient and

family report they can afford, and the prescription for that insulin is electronically transmitted to the patient's pharmacy, including any prior authorization request required. The hospitalist may have to adjust insulin dosing based upon which affordable insulin is chosen.

V. Before the patient departs the hospital for home, the discharge planning team confirms filling of the insulin prescription and the cost to the patient.

Notice how that scenario follows the primary factors and principles of capitalism. The consumer (patient) is offered all the available choices, including price transparency, then the consumer (patient) decides which choice is best based upon cost, availability, and quality. And the physician continues to manage the medical quality of care as the physician agrees to the choice decided with the patient before transmitting a prescription to a pharmacy.

MORE COMPETITION WITH LESS DISRUPTION

American healthcare can become a truer capitalistic marketplace with better consumer choice. And transitioning to a more capitalistic healthcare marketplace would minimize disruption by retaining all these current characteristics:

A. Providers retain the freedom of participating, or not, in any given healthcare insurance plan.

B. Insurance companies continue providing Medicare supplemental insurance coverage. An advantage for insurance companies would be that every American becomes a potential customer, especially once insurance companies compete across state lines. Insurance companies would also continue to offer coverage for persons present within the USA, but not eligible for Medicare coverage, such as foreign students, tourists, and other legal visitors.

C. The current computerized reimbursement infrastructure remains intact. Medicare, healthcare providers and insurance plans all continue utilizing the computer programs and systems already operating for claims, billing, and payments.

D. No wholesale elimination of a commercial enterprise. Insurance companies are also employers providing a necessary services and resources to government, providers, and consumers. Insurance companies would need to reorganize internally as they accommodate the changes with coverages and contracts and enrollments.

TAX REDUCTIONS AND BENEFITS

Yes, I propose increasing taxes. However, Americans pay approximately 18% of GDP towards healthcare regardless of any financing and reimbursement changes. So, increasing taxes towards Medicare For All must result in a reciprocal reduction of taxes and healthcare premiums elsewhere. I anticipate these other tax reductions and financial benefits from Medicare For All taxes:

- Lowered state taxes collected towards Medicaid coverage because states cover only 20% of Medicare-covered services for Medicaid-eligible residents.
- Lowered federal income taxes because income taxes currently collected to pay for Medicaid fees that would be covered by Medicare instead, rather than from being paid from income and other taxes.
- Employers realize lower per-employee benefit costs because they no longer directly pay for 100% of health insurance coverage and only pay for 20% of coverage instead. Plus, for veterans, employers would have zero direct costs for health insurance.
- Lowered automobile and workers compensation premiums. The costs of acute medical care by automobile and workers compensation insurance or would be limited to the 20% not covered by Medicare. Medicare becomes primary for all health

insurance coverage in the USA and the with elimination of the current secondary payer rules. States may offer the option for employers to cover worker injury medical costs not covered by Medicare by either participating in a state-sponsored supplemental plan or a private insurance supplemental plan. Insurance plans would freely compete on price, coverage, and quality with state-sponsored plans.

- Increased efficiency of processing and approving payment of covered services. By eliminating the secondary payer rules, Medicare would repurpose those staff currently tasked with resolving Medicare secondary payment problems to other endeavors.

- Administrative simplification at all levels of the health care system results in cost savings for all stakeholders. Physicians and other providers no longer experience significant reimbursement delays due to Medicare secondary payer enforcement. Medicare coverage guidelines apply to all Americans and eliminate the varied coverage guidelines currently existing between different health insurance plans. Providers become accountable to only one set of coverage standards, rather than several.

- A consistent and reliable appeals process for all Americans reduces administrative costs because consumers and providers access the same appeals process throughout the nation.

MODIFYING CAPITALISM

Since converting to socialism results in some awfully bad outcomes, how do we solve the problem of creating a healthcare system that enjoys the benefits of capitalism and replaces the current system of nonsense that is American healthcare?

The current economisms are feudalism, socialism, statism, capitalism, communism, and welfare state. The Peoples Republic of China is developing a hybrid economism that merges communism with capitalism. But a huge problem with communism, and the economic hybrid being developed in China, is the strong suppression of individual rights and liberties, a completely unacceptable standard in American culture. And, as mentioned, the Rands already admit that current American economics blends capitalism with socialism. In America, the healthcare services provided by the Veterans Administration is the best example of an American socialist bureaucracy.

Let us begin with a new word. I propose the word "collaborism." What is collaborism? Collaborism is an economic system where the higher classes willingly share wealth and resources with the less wealthy classes in a way that provides for the common needs of all citizens while preserving the positive attributes of capitalism, promoting wealth acquisition, personal freedom, and fair and free markets.

I predict collaborism will be the socioeconomic model for the future, and there are already many examples of collaborism already at work throughout the world. Some examples:

- Numerous nonprofit corporations and foundations exist throughout the USA and the world. Individuals and corporations make charitable donations funding the programs of the charities, and volunteers contribute to the labor force of the organization by sharing their skills and talents and reducing the labor costs for the charity.
- Charities merge with each other reducing administrative costs and retaining the ability to continue to provide essential community services despite rising expenses. For example, the Central Ohio Diabetes Association and The Columbus Cancer Clinic in Columbus, Ohio, merged into LifeCare Alliance, a non-profit that also provides meals-on-wheels, home health care and community dining centers. The mergers allow the programs assisting cancer and diabetes patients and providing cancer screening services to continue uninterrupted in a more efficient manner.
- Publicly traded corporations collaborate as multiple investors contribute their monies towards achievement of the corporations' business objectives. Corporations including stock options as part

of the compensation for their workers have already evolved to a level of collaborism. The workers share in the rewards of productivity and success both presently and in the future.

- Condominium and cooperative housing, and other fractional real estate ownership schemes such as time-shares improve secondary residence efficiency by dividing the purchase and maintenance cost of vacation properties between several or many participants.

- The interstate highway system in the USA constructed and maintained by federal fuel taxes distributed to the states. The 50 states share responsibility for a portion of the construction costs. The federal government provides nationwide transportation system oversight, while the states are responsible for the actual construction and maintenance of the highways. Everyone operating a fuel-consuming motor vehicle contributes to the cost, and all legal drivers enjoy access to the highways throughout the nation.

EXPANDED COLLABORISM

Medicare For All, under the version I propose, greatly expands a new socioeconomic system by retaining the key advantages and tempering the negative aspects of capitalism while avoiding the awful results of socialism. Collaboristic Medicare For All will possess all these attributes:

- All American citizens and legal residents share the same minimum healthcare coverage benefit throughout all the states and territories of the USA. American territories include overseas military bases and installations.

- All American citizens and legal residents contribute to the financial stability and success of the basic standard healthcare benefit.

- All American citizens and legal residents of the USA enjoy equal access to healthcare providers throughout the nation.

- All American citizens share and accept responsibility for success and accountability of Medicare coverage. All Americans are vigilant for fraudulent and abusive healthcare practices and hold elected politicians and appointed government officials accountable for operating an equitable and fair bureaucracy.
- Private enterprise and corporations accept an increased tax burden in exchange for overall lower labor costs related to healthcare insurance.
- Private healthcare plans offer balanced and fair benefits and are good stewards of the tax dollars paid to cover healthcare services. Insurance company executive compensation is reasonable and not excessive.
- All American citizens, employers, politicians, bureaucrats, health insurance plans understand and appreciate that success of Medicare For All depends on shared cooperation between and among every person and business entity in the nation. All Americans benefit because all Americans contribute.

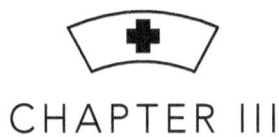

CHAPTER III

MEDICARE FOR ALL: X=Y

X=Y

The formula for financing Medicare For All begins with the simplest equation in algebra: X equals Y. Expanding on this simple equation includes details of calculating the components of both X and Y, demonstrating how X already equals Y, and the inefficient, ineffective, and inequitable methods of financing healthcare in the USA.

WHAT IS X?

The value of X is the total expenditure for healthcare services in the United States of America. In 2017, the total National Health Expenditure (NHE) in the USA was $3,492,100,000,000. Yup, that is 3.492 trillion dollars. The NHE includes all these payers and providers:

- Medicare A, B and D
- Medicare Advantage (MA) plans such as HMOs, PPOs, PSOs, and PFFS
- Prescription drug coverage
- Private employer and personal health insurance
- State Medicaid programs
- Veterans Affairs other government programs
- Home health services

- Durable medical equipment
- Dental services
- Physician and other health professions services
- Inpatient care
- Nursing home and long-term care
- Government administration
- Health insurance premiums
- Medical research

Let us further simplify all those factors into a workable method. The following abbreviations designate each classification of health care expense or payer:

- MC = All Medicare-paid services including Parts A, B, D and MA plans.
- MD = All state Medicaid plans.
- PI = All private health insurance plans.
- GOV = All other government health care financing that is not VA, MC, or MD, such as the Indian Health Service and state and local health departments.
- VA = Healthcare provided by the Veterans Administration. This does not include VA services such a burial in national cemeteries or disability payments.
- RE = Healthcare research.
- OP = Out-of-pocket expenses such as copays, coinsurance, and deductibles.

Many providers excluded from the abbreviation list such as home health, hospice, medical equipment, and others are not listed as they are reimbursed by one of the payer sources. And, this equation is about healthcare financing, not provision of care.

Therefore, the value of X expands to:

$$X = MC + MD + PI + GOV + VA + RE.$$

And keeping the equation in balance:

$$X = MC + MD + PI + GOV + VA + RE = Y.$$

Although this increases the complexity of the equation, specifying these various factors allows adjusting and manipulating the equation to understand and predict healthcare expenses and hold the various involved persons and entities accountable for assuring healthcare is sufficiently funded, and unnecessary expense and waste is reduced and avoided.

WHAT IS Y?

Y is the sources of revenue paying for healthcare services and healthcare insurance plans administration, which I abbreviate as NHR for National Healthcare Revenue. These are all the current sources of healthcare financing:

- The Medicare payroll tax paid by employers and employees.
- Health care premiums paid by employers and individuals.
- Federal and state income taxes used to pay for healthcare for veterans, state Medicaid programs and other government-funded healthcare.
- Out-of-pocket coinsurance and copay expenses.

Notice the unfairness that only income taxes, payroll taxes and health insurance premiums financially support healthcare services in the U.S.A., especially when considering how alcohol abuse, nicotine abuse, sodium and sugar and high fructose corn syrup consumption, and exposure to a wide variety of toxins contributes to healthcare needs and therefore healthcare expenses. Cigarette smoking causes cancers, but smokers avoid directly paying for the privilege of polluting their own bodies and the bodies of bystanders. Salt, added to innumerable processed foods contributes to disease such as high blood pressure, heart attacks and strokes, but also does not directly contribute to defraying the cost of the medical problems they impose. Sugars and high fructose corn syrup contribute to the occurrence of diabetes but also fail to contribute the cost of treating illness.

These abbreviations describe the current sources of healthcare funding:

- PX = Payroll taxes. PXe = Payroll tax paid by employers and PXw = Payroll tax paid by workers. Therefore PX = PXe + PXw.
- PR = Healthcare insurance premiums.
- IT = Income taxes.
- OP = Out-of-pocket expenses.

Therefore, currently: PX + PR + IT + OP = Y.
And the entire current equation is:

$$X = MC + MD + PI + GOV + VA + RE =$$

$$PX + PR + IT + OP = Y.$$

Limiting funding of healthcare to so few sources, explains the unpopularity of changing the funding method. Americans already feel they are taxed enough and charged too much for health insurance premiums. For Medicare For All to be successful, additional taxation schemes must be developed. For all of us to accept the additional taxes required to properly fund M4A, I believe the tax burden must be shared among all citizens, corporations, and employers. Industries such as food processers, nicotine products manufacturers and other toxin producers must begin paying a portion towards the cost of the healthcare illnesses their products cause.

I anticipate some may have difficulty fully understanding the formula. To hopefully simply, clarify and better visualize the formula, here is a hierarchy grid showing the components and relationships of each portion of X and each portion of Y.

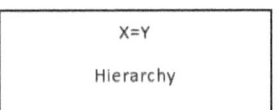

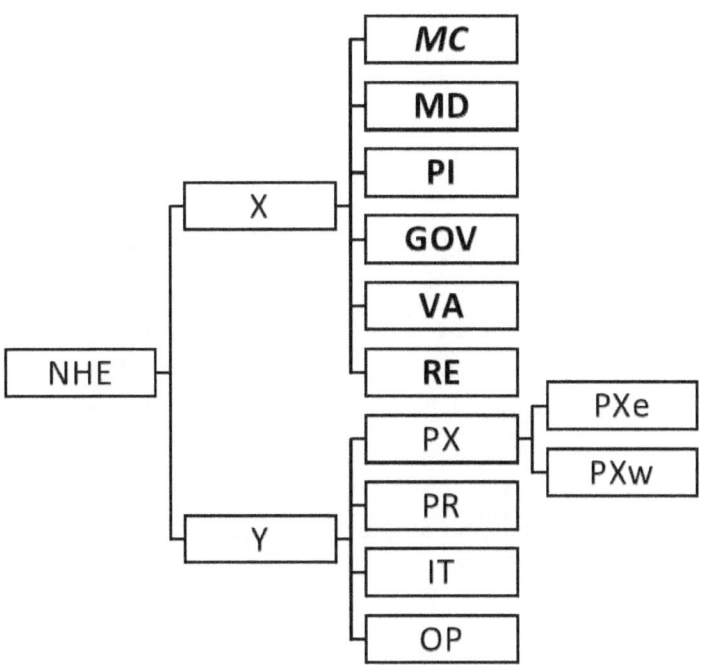

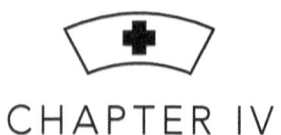

CHAPTER IV

MEDICARE FOR ALL AND TAXES

TAX REVENUE

The time has arrived for filling those algebraic values with actual numbers. And let us also revisit the issue of the limited tax resources currently financing healthcare in the United States. A significant unfairness of the current taxation system is how factors not contributing to health risks are a basis for taxation, while numerous factors contributing to health risk do not contribute to the healthcare reimbursement tax base. This chapter is written for the math geeks and policy wonks who enjoy and thrive on data analysis and mathematical computation. For those not mathletes, this chapter may be boring. However, I feel it essential including the details of my calculations, so everyone shares the faith of my diligent research, computation, and accountability. It is crucial for me that all Americans perceive my proposals and calculations and being factual, reliable, and valid.

Here is my list of other health risks that should be taxed and contribute to Medicare For All funding:

- Salt (Sodium chloride)
- Sugars (Refined sugar/added sugar/high fructose corn syrup)
- Alcohol (Ethyl alcohol for human consumption)

- Nicotine (Cigarettes, cigars, tobacco in all forms, vaping)
- Air pollution from fossil fuels (Gasoline, coal, diesel, kerosene, fuel oil, etc.)
- Air pollution from internal combustion engines (Automobiles, trucks, buses, etc.)
- Industrial toxins (Ethylene dichloride, benzene, vinyl chloride, toluene, styrene, etc.)

To add each of these sources of healthcare risk to the equation, I designate these abbreviations for each:

- Salt = Na (Na is the chemical abbreviation for sodium)
- Sugar = Su
- Alcohol = EA (Ethyl alcohol)
- Nicotine = Ni
- Air pollution from fossil fuels = FF
- Air pollution from internal combustion engines = EN
- Industrial toxins (includes ammunition) = Tn

Adding these abbreviations to the formula for PX + PR + IT + OP = Y results in the longer equation of PX + PR + IT + OP + Na + Su + EA + Ni + FF + EN + Tn = Y. Plus, adding taxes on health risk contributors allows reducing the federal income tax as a revenue source for healthcare expenses, freeing Congress to lower income tax rates and/or use those income tax revenues towards national debt reduction.

Unbelievable? Impossible? Before we go further, "income taxes" requires clarification. For this formula, I am referring to "income taxes" as taxes paid on income that are not fixed payroll taxes for Medicare and Social Security benefits. Plus, I am proposing an increase of the payroll Medicare tax. "Income taxes" for this formula include taxes paid on income to the Internal Revenue Service 1040 form line 13, that fund non-Medicare reimbursed healthcare services. Hence our equation for Y now becomes: PX + PR + ~~IT~~ + OP + Na + Su + EA + Ni + FF + EN + Tn = Y. Or, PX + PR + OP + Na + Su + EA + Ni + FF + EN + Tn = Y.

Another tax injustice is how stock exchanges do not contribute to the cost of healthcare expenses. The upper classes own most corporate stock, and middle and working classes own little stock because they do not enjoy the income to afford purchasing stock and corporations have effectively reduced worker participation with pension plans that purchase stock by substituting with 401K and 403B plans instead. I propose correcting this inequity by also taxing stock trades, and I assign the abbreviation of SE for that tax. Adding the SE tax to the Y portion, the Medicare For All equation is now:

$$X = MC+MD+PI+GOV+VA+RE =$$
$$PX+PR+OP+Na+Su+EA+Ni+FF+EN+Tn+SE = Y$$

I anticipate one of the benefits of Medicare For All will be a reduction of health insurance premiums for all employers as employers will begin covering only the 20% of healthcare services not covered by Medicare. And I am seeking to maintain the current Medicare coverage of 80% for most covered healthcare services. PI (private insurance) and MD (Medicaid) will be removed from the M4A (80%X) portion of the equation because the intent of the taxation is to cover 80% of national health expenses with payroll, consumables, and toxin taxes under Medicare For All, as state Medicaid programs would exist to cover either the uncovered portion of Medicare reimbursed services, or for services that are not a part of standard Medicare coverage. Therefore, MD (Medicaid), PR (healthcare insurance premiums) with OP (out-of-pocket) will be determined to be covering 20% of total healthcare revenues, and since X equals the total healthcare costs for the nation, MC + PI will equal 20% of national healthcare expenses; (MC + PI = 20%X). In order to properly estimate taxes, we must reduce Y by 20% as taxes will be paying for 80% of total healthcare expenses. To keep the equation in balance PR and OP must be removed from the Y side of the equation; (PR + OP = 20%Y). Now, the equation being used to estimate taxes is:

$$80\%X = MC+\sout{MD+PI}+GOV+VA+RE =$$
$$PX+\sout{PR+OP}+Na+Su+EA+Ni+FF+EN+Tn+SE = 80\%Y,$$
$$Or,$$
$$80\%X = MC+GOV+VA+RE =$$
$$PX+Na+Su+EA+Ni+FF+EN+Tn+SE = 80\%Y$$

The following explanation uses additional payroll taxes and taxation on health risk contributors to fulfill the revenue needed to meet 80% of total healthcare costs. I do not explain or explore meeting the remaining 20% of healthcare costs that would be covered by private insurance or other methods such as modified state Medicaid plans. Under this version of Medicare For All, the states would be free to develop Medicaid plans or contract with private insurance plans covering the 20% of uncovered Medicare health care costs. In addition, employers would have the freedom to contract with private employers for coverage of the 20 percent.

PX = PAYROLL TAXES

The Medicare payroll tax is currently a tax of 1.45% deducted directly from each American employee's paycheck, and a 1.45% tax paid on wages by the employer. For workers earning more than $200,000, the worker only (not the employer) pays an additional 0.9% Medicare tax on that income that exceeds $200,000. I propose that the Medicare payroll tax be increased to 4% for both the employee and employer, for a total of 8% of all payroll. In 2017, the total payroll in the U.S.A. was $16,427,300,000,000.00. Yep, that is 16.427 trillion dollars. For that payroll total, the 4% paid by employees would collect $657,092,000,000.00 and the 4% paid by employers collect another $657,092,000,000.00 for a total tax revenue of $1,314,184,000,000.00. As the National Health Expenditure for 2017 was $3,492,100,000,000.00 which equals X, which also equals Y, then 8% payroll tax collects approximately 38% of the money needed to meet the Medicare coverage for all Americans. Since reading the math in narrative seems a bit much too complicated, I restate the collection of an 8% payroll tax in equation form:

$$8\%\text{Payroll Tax} = \$1,314,184,000,000.00$$
$$X = Y = \$3,492,100,000,000.00$$
$$8\%\text{Payroll Tax} \approx 38\%X \approx 38\%Y$$

In more specific terms, the 8% payroll tax would collect 38 cents of every tax dollar collected to pay for healthcare services under Medicare For All. For those checking my calculations, please remember that 20 cents of every health care dollar will be collected from insurance premiums, direct out-of-pocket payments, or whatever funding strategies the several states devise for themselves.

I propose increasing the payroll tax because the basis of payroll tax collection one of the factors contributing to healthcare need, which is namely, being alive. Existence as a living being requires at least of minimum of health maintenance care currently covered by Medicare. I acknowledge inequity exists with payroll taxes because parents do not pay more payroll tax than a single person, therefore singles are subsidizing healthcare services for children and other nonworking family members. I do not attempt correcting that inequity as I believe all adults are responsible for the care and support of all children. I believe it to be a quintessential American family value that all American adults contribute to the health and safety and development of every American child. Also please note that I do not account for or accommodate any income limits to the payroll deduction tax. The eight percent payroll tax would be collected from all employees and employers regardless of level of pay rate. It is possible to enact a graduated tax rate on payroll so that higher earners pay a higher rate than lower earners. However, doing so greatly complicates the calculation.

I expect nearly everyone will choke on increasing the payroll tax to a total of 8%. My counter argument regards the higher payroll tax as the better deal for all Americans. My employer provides 100% payment for HMO coverage, which amounts to about $750 per month, or $9000 annually. Compared to the mean annual wage in the U.S.A. of $53,490, my employer pays about 16% towards health insurance. With the current payroll taxes for Medicare (2.9% total), the cost of healthcare is approximately 18.9% of value of a paycheck. Note how close 18.9 percent is to the 18% of GDP consumed by healthcare expenditures in the USA The net Medicare tax increase would be 5.1% (8%-2.9%=5.1%), and the employer would become responsible for only 20% of healthcare costs. Since only 20% of healthcare costs need employer coverage, the 16% current cost of HMO coverage should be reduced to 3.2% (16%x0.20=3.2%). The result would be a total of 11.2% of payroll (8%+3.2%) would be required to provide full coverage by both Medicare and a supplement to Medicare, a 7.7% cost reduction! The balance of taxation to meet remaining funds needed to implement Medicare For All comes from taxing other factors contributing to healthcare needs.

I confess that I am asking for trust of my calculations with the payroll taxes because there are wide variances between the least paid and highest paid American workers. However, I do encourage that payroll and benefits managers calculate the cost savings of increasing the payroll Medicare tax in exchange for coverage of 80% of healthcare expenses.

NON-PAYROLL TAXES

Plenty of polluting industries enjoy subsidy by the American taxpayer from both tax reduction incentives and not paying any tax that directly contributes to Medicare or any state Medicaid program. The shareholders of oil, coal and chemical-producing corporations enjoy the profits from products with adverse health effects by contaminating the air, water, and soil, promoting the ingestion of poisons via breathing, eating, and drinking. I have no opposition to any of those companies extracting and processing those substances as I am also one of the consumers who want and need those products. However, I think a great injustice of American capitalism is companies contributing to health risk which are not required to share a portion of their revenues to assure health insurance coverage for those afflicted with the injuries and illnesses that are consequences of the pollution they create.

One of my principles of taxing toxins and pollutants is taxation at the point of production, so that the corporation creating the pollution is responsible for paying the tax at the production point when the pollution occurs. And, to also prevent corporations from shifting production overseas to prevent taxation, importation of those toxic products would be taxed at the point of import. And importation of a product containing toxins is taxed on the toxins contained.

NA = SALT

I am not listing the many known negative health effects of excessive ingestion of salt, chemically known as sodium chloride. But, since the negative effects of salt are so well known, it seems exceedingly unfair that salt is not taxed in a way that contributes to defraying the healthcare costs of those salt-related illnesses. That unfairness would be reduced under this tax scheme.

In the U.S.A., 57,000,000,000 grams of salt are produced annually. Since the addition of salt to foods during process results in milligram amounts on a food label, I covert that amount to 57,000,000,000,000 milligrams. But I calculate the tax on grams of salt, as I believe it will be more effective to tax salt at its point of production (the corporations), and not its point of consumption (consumers). I propose a tax of 10 cents per gram which results in a tax of 0.010¢ per mg, or $0.00010/mg. Taxing salt at the point of production instead of consumption both assures all salt production is properly taxed and provides a financial incentive for food producers to minimize the amount of salt that is added to processed foods.

While looking at the label for 18 ounces of a national branded canned soup that contains, according to the label, 850mg of sodium. Multiplying 850mg by the tax rate of $0.00010/mg results in a 0.85¢ increase in the cost of that one can of nationally branded soup. I think that a very affordable tax. The calculation for the tax on salt as expressed as the additional cost of food is:

Milligrams of sodium x $0.00010 = added cost to food.

Taxing salt at the point of production at 10¢ per gram results in a total annual tax revenue of $5,750,000,000.00. That $5.7 billion, when divided by annual National Health Expenditure, results in salt taxation contributing 0.16% of the revenue towards funding Medicare For All, hence, taxing salt results in approximately 1/6th of 1% of tax revenue collected for Medicare reimbursement.

SU = SUGARS

In the world of chemistry, sugars are numerous sweet-tasting compounds classified as saccharides. For taxation, I am targeting only the most consumed simple sugars of refined sugar and high-fructose corn syrup, which are added a multitude of processed foods. On food labels, such sugars are listed as dextrose, sucrose, fructose, galactose, lactose, and maltose. For the purposes of taxation, dextrose, sucrose, fructose, galactose, lactose, and maltose are grouped together and taxed identically to each other. I propose taxing high fructose corn syrup separately from the other sugars because of the additional potential negative health effects from that syrup.

According to the United Stated Department of Agriculture, 10,713,000 tons of sugar were delivered for human consumption in 2018. As most food labels measure the amount of sugar in grams, we convert the tons of sugar into kilograms first. One ton equals 907.18474 kilograms Therefore 10,713,000 tons x 907.18474 kilograms equals 9,718,670,119.62 kilograms of sugar. Once again, I propose taxing sugar at the point of production, and not consumption, because the intent is to tax only sugar added to foods and to not tax any of the naturally occurring sugar present in fresh foods. The calculation for taxation of the production of sugar is:

$$10,713,000 \text{ tons x } 907.18474 \text{ kg. } = 9,718,670,119.62 \text{ kg.}$$

As there are 1000 grams per kilogram, and as most food labels list sugar content in grams, we multiply the 9,718,670,119.62 kg. by 1000 with a result of 9,718,670,119,620 grams of sugar delivered annually in the U.S.A. I propose a 5¢ per kilogram (not gram) of sugar, resulting in an equivalent of 0.005¢ or $0.00005 per gram of sugar. Such a tax would add 1/10th cent (0.01¢ or $0.0001) to the cost of that same nationally branded soup that contains 2 grams of sugar per can, a very affordable tax rate.

The proposed sugar tax would claim a total of $485,933,505.98 annually in revenue, which would be 0.01% of the total tax needed to fund Medicare For All. And this tax for granular sugar production only from sources such as sugar cane and sugar beets. Also, the sugar tax would be collected from the corporation processing the sugar cane or sugar beet into granular sugar, so that the tax burden falls on the company producing the sugar for consumption, and not the farmer growing and harvesting the sugar cane and sugar beets.

Another significant and ubiquitous source of sugar in processed foods is high fructose corn syrup (HFCS). The tax on this product is not included with that of granular sugar as each are produced differently. Granular sugar is produced from sugar cane and sugar beets, while HFCS is produced from corn. Once again, we tax HFCS at point of production, rather than consumption, so that all production is equally taxed and food producers are incentivized to reduce HFCS content in their processed foods.

In 2018, the USDA reports 6,787,000 tons of HFCS were produced in the U.S.A. As most food ingredients are listed in metric amounts, 6,157,030,660 kg. of HFCS was produced in the U.S.A. in 2018 after the tons of production is multiplied by 907.18474, which is the number of kilograms in a ton. For the math geeks, I clarify that I refer to tons in America (2000 lbs.), known as a "short ton," and not to the metric tonne, which is 1000 kilograms or 2,204 pounds.

The calculation for HFCS production is:

6,787,000 tons x 907.18474 = 6,157,062,830 kg.

Food labels tend to list HFCS in grams rather than milligrams. I propose a 1/10¢ ($0.001) tax per gram, which is a $1 per kilogram tax on HFCS production. On a label for a popular cola product, a 12-ounce bottle of soda contains 69 grams of sugars. Since the same label does not mention any other sugar in the list of ingredients, the entire sugar content of that bottle of soda pop is the full 69 grams. At \$0.001 per gram, \$0.069 or 6.9¢ is added to the cost of the bottle of soda, which I believe to be an affordable price for most Americans. As a percent of contribution, such a tax on HFCS would be 0.18% towards the national health expenditure (NHE).

I acknowledge taxing HFCS at a higher rate than the tax rate for sugar. Even though there is the marketing tag line, "sugar is sugar," that is not quite accurate for high fructose corn syrup. Refined sugar is a naturally occurring compound processed and extracted from sugar beets and sugar cane. But HFCS is not a naturally occurring compound. Fructose itself is naturally occurring, but it does not occur at that concentration in nature. Corporations extract glucose from the corn in a manner inconsistent with the natural chemical structure of corn. HFCS is produced by extracting glucose from corn, then using enzymes to convert it to fructose in a concentration that does not occur in nature. A primary motive for the use of HFCS is that HFCS costs less than refined sugar to produce, thereby contributing to the profit motive of food producers. HFCS is associated with the prevalence of obesity in America as the excessive ingestion of HFCS as fructose in human livers prefers to convert fructose to fat, rather than into other sugars.

If you cut a sugar cane and suck on the end, it tastes sweet because the sugar is already there. With HFCS, if you suck on a raw piece of corn, the taste is bland because the sugar content is not freely and naturally available to your taste buds. The sugars in corn must be processed into a form that has a sweet taste. For example, sweet corn for human consumption does not taste sweet until it is cooked, and the heat of cooking releases the sugar content into a form detectable to one's taste buds.

HFCS creates its' negative health effects because of its more-rapid-than-sugar absorption from the intestine, and the chemical processing differences in the liver. Since the liver prefers to convert HFCS to fat, illnesses such as high cholesterol, non-alcoholic fatty liver and diabetes are promoted and aggravated. The other sugars, particularly glucose, trigger the release of insulin, which is the hormone that reduces blood sugar. HFCS does not trigger insulin release, thwarting the body's natural method to manage and control blood sugar levels.

An additional illness created and worsened by HFCS is gout, a type of arthritis. Gout occurs because a waste product called uric acid accumulates in the blood, which then leaches into and deposits into joint spaces, causing pain, stiffness, and inflammation. Hence, HFCS is indeed not "sugar is sugar."

EA = ALCOHOL

For purposes of tax collection towards Medicare For All expenses, alcohol refers to only ethyl alcohol for human consumption. Ethyl alcohol added to hand sanitizers, and other formulations not intended for ingestion are excluded. And, other alcohols, such a methyl alcohol, that are poisonous, or otherwise used for a manufacturing purpose are also excluded from this category. However, alcohols used for industrial production could be added to the toxins category of items taxed.

Ethyl alcohol is available in so many different forms of beers, wines, and liquors, that attempting to tax based on volume became unmanageably time consuming. As a compromise simplifying the taxation, I base the alcohol tax towards M4A on the total sales of alcohol in the USA. The most recent data indicates that $234,380,000,000 was sold in the USA. I impose and calculate a 15% tax on those sales, resulting in an annual receipt of $35,157,000,000 towards M4A funding, a 1.01% portion of M4A receipts or 0.18% of GDP.

In concede how the taxation on alcohol is high. However, I justify the tax because of the numerous well-known chronic diseases linked to alcohol abuse, such as fatty liver, liver cirrhosis and diabetes. Those illnesses inflict many years of suffering and high healthcare expenses. Plus, alcohol consumption is voluntary as one can chose to drink or not drink alcohol.

NI = NICOTINE PRODUCTS

The subsidy provided to nicotine-containing products is truly phenomenal when one considers all the negative and chronic medical impacts to individuals and society. Previously, we would have discussed tobacco products. However, with the advent of e-cigarettes that do not contain any actual tobacco, we focus on the common minimal ingredient of that most addictive of substances—nicotine. Nicotine-containing substances are responsible for a long list of cancers, lung disease, heart disease and intestinal disease that afflicts not only the direct consumer of the product, but also the bystander inhaling the smoke or vaper in the air. And yet, there is no direct federal tax on nicotine-containing products towards covering the high medical costs of those afflictions.

SMOKELESS TOBACCO

Smokeless tobacco includes products such as snuff and chewing tobacco. In 2018, the Federal Trade Commission report 128,405,325 pounds of smokeless tobacco were sold in the USA. Since there appears to be a variety of weights of the tins of smokeless tobacco between the various brands, I also chose taxing smokeless tobacco at the point of production, rather than the point of consumption. Imposing a tax of $5 per pound results in an annual tax revenue of $642,026,625.00, which is 0.02% of the revenue needed to fund Medicare For All.

CIGARETTES

According to data published by the Federal Trade Commission, 229,100,000,000 cigarettes were sold in the USA in 2017, which fortunately is a declining statistic. I propose a tax of 50¢ per cigarette, which would greatly increase the price of a pack of cigarettes. A half-dollar tax per cigarette would result in an annual tax revenue of $114,550,000,000.00. The 114.55 billion dollars of revenue contributes only 3.28% towards the total annual cost of Medicare For All. I have little sympathy for those complaining about high taxation of cigarettes, because cigarette smoke not only poisons the air of the smoker, it also poisons the air of bystanders and cigarette butts contaminate the ground. Cigarettes are toxic to all life forms regardless of purchaser.

CIGARS

Cigar taxation requires a calculation adjustment because much of cigar production occurs in foreign countries, meaning most cigars are imported. Hence, I devise a taxing strategy where all cigar production is equally taxed eliminating any advantage or disadvantage to producing cigars within or outside the USA. In 2017, the cigar market in the USA was 13,047,000,000 pieces. I do not differentiate between domestic-produced or foreign-produced cigars and tax both equally at 25¢ per piece, which generates $3,261,750,000.00 in annual revenue for Medicare For All. Taxing at point of production or import assures that the tax contribution is collected regardless of sales. Cigars stored on a market shelf or in a warehouse have already been taxed and the vendor can determine how to cover the cost of the additional tax by adjusting the sales price if they wish.

VAPING

In 2017, 121,082,297 e-cigarette units were sold in the USA. I propose charging 10¢ per unit as a standard tax, in addition to whatever sales or other taxes are already collected and assigning that 10 cents per unit tax to funding Medicare For All, which results in $12,108,229.70 being collected annually towards Medicare For All.

HYDROCARBONS

Hydrocarbons, primarily the fuels of gasoline, diesel, kerosene, fuel oil and coal, contribute to illness and injury via air pollution generated by the combustion of those substances, and via ground and water pollution from their byproducts. For example, the combustion of coal results in the creation of coal ash, which is stored in ponds on or near the locations of coal-fired electric power plants. The coal ash contaminates and poisons the surrounding land and water, especially when an ash pond becomes overflowing, such as during heavy rains. I use the abbreviation EN to distinguish those hydrocarbons combusted in an engine, and the abbreviation FF identifying those hydrocarbons combusted in furnaces.

I propose taxing hydrocarbons both at point of production and combustion. In other words, additional taxes would be added at the point of production, and during use. For coal, taxation would occur upon mining, and for the other fuels, upon production at a refinery. The option exists to tax fuels at the point of consumption by imposing the tax when the gasoline is pumped into a motor vehicle, or kerosene is pumped into an airplane fuel tank. However, I am in favor of taxation at point of production so that the distributor and retailer bear the burden of tax collection regardless of the price of the fuel.

For gasoline, I propose a 15¢ per gallon tax, for diesel a 30¢ per gallon tax and for kerosene used for jet fuel, a 50¢ per gallon tax. I do not propose a tax on kerosene utilized for heating only because I was unable to locate a reliable source of data regarding the production and use of kerosene for heating.

For fuel oil residual and distillates, I calculate a 20¢ per gallon tax for both. And for coal, I add a $200 per ton tax to be collected upon extraction from the mine.

Annually, collected at point of registration renewal, an additional $75 per personal vehicle tax collection for motor vehicles that are not SUVs, pickups, semi-trucks or buses. For SUVs and pickups, the annual tax increases to $125 each; for semi-trucks a $1000 per vehicle tax is imposed, and for each bus, collection of an annual $3000.

In the following table, I list each of the EN and FF items, anticipated tax receipts and percentage of GDP gleaned by each tax rate. Please note that the percentage of GDP is equivalent to the number of cents per dollar spent in the U.S.A., so the total collected for personal vehicles is only 1/10 of one cent.

	Source	Receipt	%GDP
EN	Gasoline	$ 16,084,778,850.00	0.08%
EN	Diesel-on highway	$ 12,421,500,000.00	0.06%
EN	Kerosene Jet	$ 3,850,000,000.00	0.02%
FF	Fuel Oil-Residual	$ 638,000.00	0.000003%
FF	Fuel Oil-Distillate	$ 12,469,400,000.00	0.06%
FF	Coal	$ 151,104,600,000.00	0.77%
EN	Vehicle-Personal	$ 19,224,327,075.00	0.10%
EN	Vehicle-SU Trucks	$ 1,093,314,750.00	0.01%
EN	Vehicle-Semi	$ 2,752,043,000.00	0.01%
EN	Buses	$ 2,928,483,000.00	0.02%

FIREARMS AND AMMUNITION

Firearms are another business subsidized by not requiring a tax contribution to the health problems associated with their use. Bullets cannot inflict bodily damage by themselves and require being discharged at high velocities from a combustion chamber. And bullets tearing through flesh, bone, muscle, and internal organs sufficiently explains the impact of ammunition on healthcare. I classify ammunition as an industrial toxin both because of the physical trauma inflicted by the penetration of ammunition into a human body, and the heavy metals, such as lead, that leach into blood and body fluids inflicting additional stress and chemical trauma to organs and body structures.

An interesting problem encountered while researching firearms and ammunition production was the great difficulty locating a reliable source of production data for both. However, I able to locate a report from the National Shooting Sports Foundation, Inc. listing the taxes paid by the firearms industry in 2018 was $3,965,700,800 in federal business taxes and $653,764,800 in excise taxes. I was not able to discern or separate how much of either tax was paid for ammunition or firearms with the other production taxes, I focus on taxation of production, not consumption, but in the case of firearms and ammunition, I decided simply to transfer the already collected federal business taxes to Medicare

For All funding. If readily available (read: "free") information about ammunition and firearm production becomes available on the internet, I will happily revise the calculation. Until then, the federal business taxes are already collected and would simply be redirected within the federal budget to contribute to Medicare For All funding.

OTHER TOXINS

A wide variety of industrial toxins are produced in the USA each year. However, listing and taxing every toxin would generate an extremely long list. Hence, I limit taxation to those classifications of toxins that are both frequently produced, and for which I was able to identify reliable production data. The data for each is reported in pounds, so the tax imposed at point of production is also per pound. Organophosphate producers would pay a tax of $25 per pound, while the producers of ethylene dichloride, benzene, vinyl chloride, toluene and styrene would incur a tax of $10 per pound for each toxin. As with the hydrocarbons, this grid lists each toxin, the anticipated annual receipts for each tax, and the percentage of GDP for each.

	Source	Receipt	%GDP
Tn	Organophosphates	$ 500,000,000.00	0.0026%
Tn	Ethylene dichloride	$ 280,000,000,000.00	1.43%
Tn	Benzene	$ 237,000,000,000.00	1.21%
Tn	Vinyl chloride	$ 167,000,000,000.00	0.86%
Tn	Toluene	$ 151,000,000,000.00	0.77%
Tn	Styrene	$ 102,000,000,000.00	0.52%

SE = STOCK EXCHANGES

Although stock ownership does not have a direct relationship with healthcare risk, other than ownership of stock in companies that produce toxic products, I include a taxation on stock exchanges because stock ownership exemplifies the great disparity of wealth distribution in America. Barry Ritholtz of Ritholtz Wealth Management, LLC reports these comparisons:

1. Only half of Americans own equities either directly, or indirectly via a pension plan.
2. 10% of Americans own 84% of all stocks.

Although some argue against stocks taxation, I disagree because those same publicly traded corporations will enjoy lesser labor costs once M4A is fully implemented, which could improve their stock performance. In addition, the savings from the lowered labor costs eventually enriches the bottom line of those corporations and improves the ability to pay stock dividends to the shareholders.

Approximately 6,430,000,000 stocks are traded per day, and stock exchanges are open 252 days per year (365 days, minus weekends, minus nine observed holidays, equals 252). I propose taxing each share of stock traded at 10¢ ($0.10). Multiplying 6,430,000,000 stocks per day x 10¢ for each stock x 252 days results in $162,036,000,000.00 annual tax revenue in support of M4A which is 4.64% of the taxation needed to fund M4A, or 0.83% of GDP, or less than 1¢ of every dollar spent in America. Although I anticipate stockholders and traders will cry foul to this proposal, I further explore capitalism, and improving and enhancing capitalism in another chapter.

The spreadsheet created calculating and summing all the proposed Medicare For All taxes is quite extensive, therefore in the interest of transparency, here is the full spreadsheet:

Classification		Source	Tax	Base/2017		Receipt	Now	% goal	%GDP
Payroll	PXw	Medicare employee	4.00%	$16,427,300,000,000.00		$657,092,000,000.00	1.45%		
Taxes	PXe	Medicare employer	4.00%	$16,427,300,000,000.00		$657,092,000,000.00	1.45%		
	PX	Total Payroll	8.00%	$16,427,300,000,000.00		$1,314,184,000,000.00	2.90%	37.63%	6.73%
	Su	Sugar	$ 0.05	9,718,670,119.62	Kg	$ 485,933,505.98		0.01%	0.0025%
Consumables	Su	HF Corn Syrup	$ 1.000	6,157,062,830.38	Kg	$ 6,157,062,830.38		0.18%	0.03%
	Na	Salt	$ 0.10	57,000,000,000	Gm	$ 5,700,000,000.00		0.16%	0.03%
	EA	Alcohol	15%	$ 234,380,000,000.00	$	$ 35,157,000,000.00		1.01%	0.18%
	Ni	Smokeless Tobacco	$ 5.00	128,405,325	lbs	$ 642,026,625.00		0.02%	0.0033%
Nicotine	Ni	Annual cigarettes	$ 0.50	229,100,000,000	per	$ 114,550,000,000.00		3.28%	0.59%
Products	Ni	Cigars	$ 0.25	13,047,000,000	per	$ 3,261,750,000.00		0.0934%	0.0167%
	Ni	Vaping	$ 0.10	121,082,297	per	$ 12,108,229.70		0.0003%	0.0001%
	EN	Gasoline	$ 0.15	107231859000.00	gal	$ 16,084,778,850.00		0.46%	0.08%
	EN	Diesel-on hwy	$ 0.30	41,405,000,000.00	gal	$ 12,421,500,000.00		0.36%	0.06%
	EN	Kerosene Jet	$ 0.50	7,700,000,000	gal	$ 3,850,000,000.00		0.11%	0.02%
	FF	Fuel Oil-Residual	$ 0.20	3,190,000,000	gal	$ 638,000,000.00		0.000018%	0.000003%
Hydrocarbons	FF	Fuel Oil-Distillate	$ 0.20	62,347,000,000	gal	$ 12,469,400,000.00		0.36%	0.06%
	FF	Coal	$ 200.00	755,523,000	ton	$ 151,104,600,000.00		4.33%	0.77%
	EN	Vehicle-Personal	$ 75.00	256,324,361.00	per	$ 19,224,327,075.00		0.55%	0.10%
	EN	Vehicle-SU Trucks	$ 125.00	8,746,518.00	per	$ 1,093,314,750.00		0.03%	0.01%
	EN	Vehicle-Semi	$ 1,000.00	2,752,043.00	per	$ 2,752,043,000.00		0.08%	0.01%
	EN	Buses	$ 3,000.00	976,161.00	per	$ 2,928,483,000.00		0.08%	0.02%
	Tn	Firearms & Ammo		$ 3,965,700,800.00	$	$ 3,965,700,800.00		0.1136%	0.0203%
				Industrial Toxins					
	Tn	Organophosphates	$ 25.00	20,000,000	Lbs	$ 500,000,000.00		0.01%	0.0026%
Toxins	Tn	Ethylene dichloride	$ 10.00	28,000,000,000.00	Lbs	$ 280,000,000,000.00		8.02%	1.43%
	Tn	Benzene	$ 10.00	23,700,000,000.00	Lbs	$ 237,000,000,000.00		6.79%	1.21%
	Tn	Vinyl chloride	$ 10.00	16,700,000,000.00	Lbs	$ 167,000,000,000.00		4.78%	0.86%
	Tn	Toluene	$ 10.00	15,100,000,000.00	Lbs	$ 151,000,000,000.00		4.32%	0.77%
	Tn	Styrene	$ 10.00	10,200,000,000.00	Lbs	$ 102,000,000,000.00		2.92%	0.52%
Stock exchange	SE	Stock trade	$ 0.10	6,430,000,000	day	$ 162,036,000,000.00	252	4.64%	0.83%
		Total receipts:				$2,805,580,666,666.06		100.43%	14.37%
		NHE 2017				$3,492,100,000,000.00			17.89%
		Goal:		NHE 2017 x 80%		$2,793,680,000,000.00			
		GDP 2017				$19,519,400,000,000.00			
		HI premiums		NHE x 20%		$698,420,000,000.00	9.10		0.035780813
				Per person HI premium	yr	2,134.75			
				Per person HI premium	mo	177.90			

EASIER MATH

The problem with big numbers, is just that they are big numbers and difficult to recall and understand. To make it easier for all to better understand how the tax proposals will properly fund Medicare For All, I now convert the tax collected into a percentage of gross domestic product (GDP). As I use the year 2017 for the National Health Expenditure, I also use the GDP for 2017 so the comparisons are as similar as possible. According to countryeconomy.com, the GDP for the U.S.A. in 2017 $19,519,400,000,000.00. Yep, that is over 19 trillion American dollars!

The spreadsheet itself is quite detailed, and wonderful for math and accounting geeks, but not so useful for everyone else. I do include the spreadsheet though because I desire following the common grade school admonition of "show your work." And another great value of the spreadsheet regards the flexibility of the formula. When production of a taxed item decreases, or the tax receipts on any taxed item declines, the formula itself is preserved, allowing upward adjustment of other taxed items to compensate for any potential funding deficiency. Also, any additional ideas for taxable items may be easily added to the spreadsheet, and calculation.

To further simply and provide a better visual, I include here a hierarchy of the tax structure and formula. This graphic represents the formula itself without the breakdown of costs and revenues.

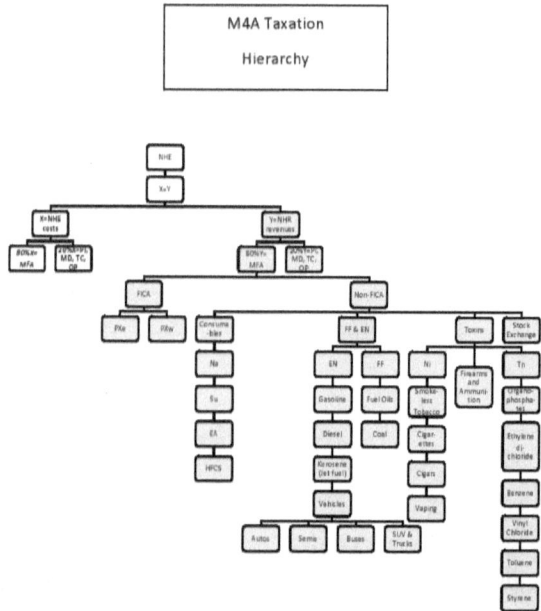

Since converting the annual tax collection for each taxable item as a percentage of GDP allows expressing the tax rate as a portion of each dollar spent in the USA, converting into a percentage of GDP allows me to represent the total GDP as one dollar, and then represent each annual tax collection as the number of cents of each dollar spent in the USA. I am confident most will agree that viewing the tax rates as a portion of each dollar makes it much easier to understand how the taxation affects your wallet.

Using a percentage of GDP calculation allows me to first express that since the National Healthcare Expenditure is approximately 17.89% of GDP, then approximately 18¢ of each American dollar is spent on healthcare. And, since I am attempting to only fund the 80% coverage of healthcare costs with taxes, that results needing tax revenues of 14.31¢ of each GDP dollar to meet the funding requirements for Medicare For All (17.89¢ x 0.8 [80%] =14.31¢). Please recall how currently approximately 18¢ of every American dollar is spent on healthcare regardless if Medicare For All is enacted or not. The change I propose with my version of M4A assures more equitable distribution of the 18¢ spent on healthcare among all Americans and greatly reduces the current cost and quality of care discrepancies between races and social classes.

On the spreadsheet, I listed each tax category and item, the proposed tax rate, the percentage of coverage of Medicare For All funding and the percentage of Gross Domestic Product. The percentage of goal reveals which percentage of NHE is covered by that tax. Since the goal is to fund 80% of NHE, I need the total percentage from all collected taxes to equal 100%. I list this only to demonstrate how I have indeed devised a tax structure that would fund Medicare For All at the current level of Medicare covering 80% of allowed health care services, drugs, devices, and products. The more important column is the %GDP. I converted the tax collected to a percentage of GDP, so an easy comparison can be made to each dollar spent in the American economy. So, in the GDP column %=¢. Therefore, of every dollar spent in America, 6.73 cents fund the payroll tax contribution for Medicare For All. Notice how incrementally small some of the taxation rates are when compared as a percentage of GDP. Several percentages had to be expanded to 4 places past the decimal point, and one was expanded to 6 places past the decimal point, otherwise, if rounded at only 2 spaces past the decimal point, those percentages would display as 0.00%.

And please notice at the bottom of the spreadsheet how I exceed the requirement for full funding of Medicare For All. Converted to dollars and cents as a percentage of GDP, the taxing scheme collects 14.34%, or 14.34¢ per dollar of GDP per year, exceeding the required 14.31% or 14.31¢ per dollar of GDP. Next is the same funding hierarchy, with the cents-per-GDP dollar added to each taxed item, which should provide a better visual regarding how each taxed item contributes to the total M4A funding.

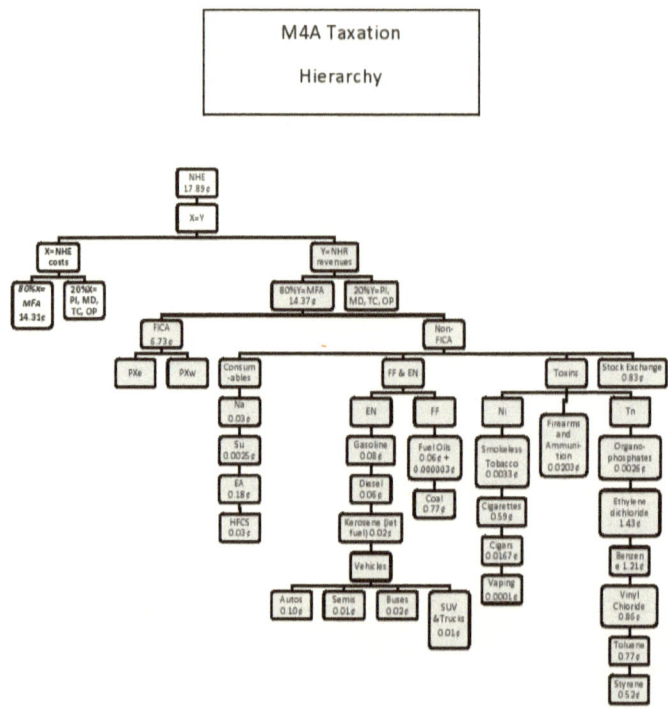

So hopefully every reader and American citizen now understands and appreciates how Medicare For All funding is both possible, and affordable.

TAXING PRINCIPLES

Although some of the taxation principles as I described were explained with each taxable item, I list them here for further clarity. I think it essential all Americans feel the taxes are fair and reasonable. Here is the list of the principles of taxation:

1. All taxes collected are assigned for Medicare reimbursement of health care charges and applicable and reasonable administrative expenses to provide reimbursement. The Congressional Budget Office refers to this as "earmarking." Tax assignment reduces the ability of Congress, a Presidential administration, or the courts from altering or manipulating funding of Medicare For All.
2. For payroll taxes, everyone pays the same rate. No worker is exempted from the payroll tax and all payroll is taxed.
3. Wherever possible, products taxed are taxed at point of production, not consumption. And point of importation equals the point of production for those products manufactured outside the USA.
4. Factors that contribute to healthcare need and cost are taxed, eliminating the current indirect subsidy of toxic chemical production.
5. Taxes collected should approximately equal 80% of the total National Health Expenditure so that there is a reasonable comparison.
6. No political bribes or poison pills—I do not offer or promote any additional healthcare service coverage beyond that which is already covered by Medicare. But I do advocate eliminating all Medicare secondary payer rules so that Medicare becomes the primary healthcare payer for all Americans in all domestic healthcare situations. I also do not delve into the political quagmire of attempting to fund abortions. I strive for my version of M4A to be appealing to the many and objectionable to the few.

TAXATION STRENGTHS AND WEAKNESSES

All ideas and schemes have strengths and weaknesses. I list them here for better communication about my awareness of them and to allow others further analysis and constructive criticism of the taxation scheme. The strengths of my proposed taxes are:

- As many contributing factors to healthcare needs and costs contributes directly towards healthcare funding.
- The scheme is flexible: Providing total percentages of GDP are preserved, taxable categories can be added or eliminated, and taxation amounts can be negotiated and adjusted. A reduction or elimination of one tax category can be compensated with either and additional tax category or increase of taxation of one or more of the other categories.
- All Americans contribute and all Americans benefit. Social inequalities of healthcare access and reimbursement are greatly reduced.
- Total labor costs are reduced for employers and those reductions are paid by taxation of toxins.
- Veterans and active military are 100% covered for Medicare-reimbursed services and retain those benefits without additional direct expense to any employer.
- Basic healthcare coverage for every American is no longer enslaved to employment. Layoffs and other job terminations result in a loss of Medicare supplement coverage only.
- Congress, Presidential administrations, and the courts lose the ability to use Medicare taxes for any other purpose.
- The calculations are evidenced based as anyone with internet access and basic algebra education can verify the calculations, propose alternatives and adjustments, and detect and report errors and miscalculations.
- There is something for everyone to like. Every American would enjoy basic Medicare coverage regardless of employment or social status. All employers would enjoy a reduction of total

labor costs and every state and territory would realize a reduction of funding burden for Medicaid programs.

- There are many choices and options available. I intentionally offer as many options as possible both as persuasion for my fellow Americans to adopt my ideas, but also allowing and promoting maximum pliability so that nearly every unusual employment and social situation can be accommodated.

And now the list of weaknesses:

- There is something for everyone to dislike. Average American workers and employers will dislike the proposed increasing of payroll taxes and stockholders will dislike the proposed tax on each stock exchange. Toxin producers will oppose the taxes on their products and food processors will object to the taxes on salt, sugar, and high fructose corn syrup.
- The data is not real-time. Calculating on current data would be wonderful, but accessibility to such data is another question. I worked to assure that all data used was the most current and freely available on the internet so that any American can fact-check and verify both sources and calculations.
- Political realities are intentionally disregarded. I demonstrate an achievable, sound, and distributed taxation policy and law. This book is about reliable mathematical calculation, not political accommodation. I desire a dialogue with all Americans, not just the political and business elite.
- Implementation requires courage and lots of it. American voters would need to demand government representatives enact the legal and taxation changes and hold providers, politicians, bureaucrats, and insurance plans accountable. State and federal bureaucracy would need to adapt on an extended basis a different mode of operation. Insurance companies would adapt their operations and fees to accommodate providing of Medicare supplemental or Medicare Advantage plans.

- Implementation requires patience, and plenty of it. The tax scheme will require gradual and progressive implementation preventing shocks to the economy. Enrollment will require progressive, prioritized implementation so that the Social Security Administration is not overwhelmed with the enrollment process.

- Mathematics always includes errors and inaccuracies, and my tax proposal is no exception. For the calculations to be understood by most Americans, results have been rounded for simplicity. Anyone offering a more accurate calculation are free to share their revision.

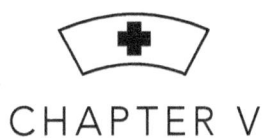

CHAPTER V

MEDICARE FOR ALL AND PRIVATE INSURANCE

WHY END PRIVATE INSURANCE?

Some politicians and others promoting Medicare For All demand termination of all private health insurance with replacement by government-managed healthcare. What a lousy idea! The primary argument against health insurance corporations is their history of mismanagement and abuse and disregard for patient needs. In an ideal world, that would be a wonderful concept. Unfortunately, as I explain in the chapter about politics and economisms, it is a bad idea because substituting with a socialistic system also potentially results in mismanagement, abuse, and disregard for patient needs.

Mismanagement and abuse occur throughout the corporate world, but we do not demand government absorption and control of those other mismanaged corporations. Here are some examples of corporate mismanagement resulting in mistreatment of consumers:

- Volkswagen conspires and subverts the exhaust emission standards on their diesel-powered vehicles.
- Boeing fails with properly confirming the software of a new class of jet airplane operates properly, resulting in airplane crashes and multiple passenger and crew deaths.

- Oil pipeline leaks occur on a regular basis, polluting waterways, and the surrounding environment.
- Toyota manufactured automobiles with defective accelerators, resulting in collisions, injuries, and deaths.

Each example of corporate mismanagement or neglect did not result in demands that automobile manufacturers, aerospace corporations or petroleum companies be dissolved, with their operations completely assumed by a government agency. Why target health insurance corporations for destruction? However, that does not mean there is not plenty of room for improvement with health insurance company operations and practices. Here are some well publicized sins by health insurance companies:

- On December 20, 2002, the Ohio Supreme Court imposed a $32.5 million damage award against Anthem Blue Cross and Blue Shield, $30 million dollars of being for punitive damages in the case of *Dardinger vs. Anthem Blue Cross and Blue Shield.* The damages awarded compensated for the failure of the insurance plan to properly follow record review procedures regarding authorization requests for additional chemotherapy for a patient with a brain tumor. The patient died from the brain tumor and her surviving spouse sued the insurance company for breach of contract and other torts.
- In 2011, CareSource, a managed care benefits company headquartered in Dayton, OH, paid $26 million settled false claim charges where the insurance plan charged a state Medicaid program for case management services which were never provided.

One might think that both examples support the argument for eliminating health insurance companies. Please consider that while those two insurance plans failed in their duties and responsibilities, many other health insurance plans did not improperly deny needed medical care and did not cheat the federal and state government out of tax dollars, the same as while Boeing failed with proper engineering of their airliner model, the other aircraft manufacturers were assuring proper engineering. Also please consider we do not demand dismantling of the aerospace industry when an airplane crash occurs, do not demand expulsion of all politicians from office when one is found guilty of corruption, and do not demand elimination of all municipal water companies when one allows lead contamination of its water supply. We obviously recognize how large organizations provide benefits to individuals and society despite the interference from human greed, stupidity, and ignorance. We need elimination and reduction of greed, stupidity, and ignorance, not elimination of corporations.

BENEFITS OF HEALTH INSURANCE PLANS.

Health insurance plans provide many benefits for government, employers, and beneficiaries. However, the benefits may be hidden from the average consumer and may appear as mystical. It is time to demystify those benefits.

WHEELCHAIRS FOR EVERYONE?

Insurance companies, to stay financially viable, like all businesses, must have cost controls, otherwise their businesses fail because claims paid exceeds premiums received. The absence of cost controls incentivizes the temptation for false claims without a process challenging and confirming the validity of claims. Automobile insurers accomplish cost control via claims adjusters confirming actual damages overseeing proper claims payment. For health insurance, the process is known as prior authorization or "prior auth," or utilizations management or "UM." The lawsuit against Anthem Blue Cross and Blue Shield exemplifies when the prior auth procedure goes awry. Without prior authorization, physicians could prescribe any covered medical service reimbursed by insurance without restraint. We could all request prescriptions for wheelchairs for ourselves because no one would assure any actual medical need for a wheelchair. Wouldn't it be wonderful if none us had to walk anywhere because health insurance would pay for everyone's possession and use of a wheelchair? Although using the wheelchair analogy is an obvious exaggeration, it depicts the reason and necessity for prior authorization and medical review of high-cost medical procedures, medications, and devices.

For most healthcare benefits, Medicare, except through contracted Medicare Advantage plans, lacks the ability performing prior authorizations because the claims for tens of millions of covered Americans are simply too vast for timely and effective pre-payment review. Medicare utilizes alternative methods for cost controls, but the cost controls are retrospective, meaning imposition of the cost control after delivery of the medical product or service to the patient. Health insurance prior auth is prospective, that is, looking at the claim and prescription before provision or delivery to the patient. An advantage of prospective prior auth is the insurance plan confirms medical necessity for the prescribed service or item is documented in the patient's medical record before the medical provider provides the service or item to the patient. The disadvantage of prior authorization is the delay of providing the service or item to the patient until after the prior auth approval, and if the prior auth process becomes prolonged for any reason, the patient waits until correction of the prior auth process. Such situations are why health insurance plans as a group share the undesirable reputation of interfering with the provision of needed medical care to patients.

The retrospective system adopted by Medicare has the advantage of no prior auth interfering with delay of delivery of service to a patient. The disadvantage is that the medical provider takes the financial risk that Medicare will decline payment after the service or item has already been provided to the patient when medical documentation insufficiently explains the medical necessity, or other glitches during a medical record audit. Medicare's retrospective process for cost control involves cost reports, fee schedules, bundled payments and auditing strategies such as Recovery Audit Contractors.

COST REPORTS

Medical providers billing Medicare are required by law and regulation to submit periodic cost reports to Medicare explaining in detail the costs of doing business as a medical enterprise. Cost reports include items such as wages and benefits and other labor costs, office expenses such as leases, supplies and equipment and other allowed and recognized expenses incurred by medical providers. Medicare uses audited cost reports to determine reasonable reimbursement rates to medical providers. Unfortunately, a reality of cost reports is the lag time between reporting by medical providers and auditing by Medicare, as Medicare lacks the ability to audit cost reports in real-time. Hence, Medicare bases reimbursement rates on past financial data which does not easily accommodate sudden changes with medical provider operations during disasters or other situations where a sudden change of medical care demand occurs.

FEE SCHEDULES

Medicare publishes and updates extensive fee schedules listing the various types of covered medical services, and the reimbursement rates for those services. Medicare determines fee schedules amounts based on audits of cost reports.

BUNDLED PAYMENTS

Instead of paying for itemized medical services and products, for inpatient care, outpatient care, and home health, Medicare pays a bundled rate for all the services provided by the hospital, outpatient center or home health agency. An assessment of the patient's illness, medical needs and level of disability affects the reimbursement rates. More ill patients requiring more medical care result in greater bundled payment rates and vice versa. Again, Medicare bases reimbursement rates on the results of audited cost reports. Depending on the contract with Medicare, a Medicare Advantage plan may not use bundled payments.

RECOVERY AUDIT CONTRACTORS

Instead of employing teams of auditors reviewing medical records for proper payment by Medicare, CMS contracts with Recovery Audit Contractors (RACs) that provide medical record and medical claims auditing. RACs, after auditing a hospital or other medical provider, receive a portion of the money recovered by Medicare during the audit. This arrangement encourages the RAC auditors to thoroughly review medical records for every possible incorrect overpayment by Medicare. However, it also discourages RAC auditors from unnecessarily auditing medical providers compliant with documentation and Medicare claims requirements.

COVERAGE OF NON-CITIZENS

Another good reason eliminating private health insurance plans is a terrible idea concerns the intent of Medicare For All covering all American citizens and legal residents. That leaves illegal immigrants, foreigners legally present but not residents (visa holders) and other foreign visitors such as tourists needing coverage while present in the country. For example, foreign workers present in the USA under a HB-1 work visa would be excluded from coverage. Excluding such visa holders both removes any incentive and creates a disincentive for corporate displacement of American workers and replacing them foreign workers. Hiring foreign workers requires the workers and their employers pay the Medicare tax on their incomes and requires either the worker or the employer purchase separate private healthcare coverage while the worker is present in the country. As well, all foreigners present in the country not properly designated as a legal resident of America, would also be required to purchase, and provide a proof of coverage for healthcare from a private insurer.

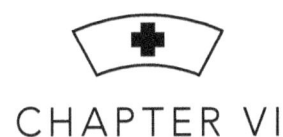

CHAPTER VI

MEDICARE FOR ALL AND THE VETERANS ADMINISTRATION

VETERANS ADMINISTRATION

I think all Americans agree on the importance of the Veterans Administration with assuring veterans receive quality healthcare, especially those veterans injured during combat. The *Merriam-Webster Dictionary* defines socialism as any of various economic and political theories advocating collective or <u>governmental ownership</u> and <u>administration</u> of the means of production. Since opponents of Medicare For All will waive the warning flag of socialism, I use the current situation with VA healthcare as a shining example of failed socialism, and how my proposal for Medicare For All eliminates the socialistic problems currently plaguing VA healthcare.

ONLY VA HEALTHCARE

My proposals to VA services under Medicare For All affect <u>only</u> healthcare services provided by the VA that are <u>also</u> Medicare-covered services. All other services and benefits, such as pensions, long term care, survivor benefits, employment assistance, housing and insurance assistance, burial and memorials would continue unchanged.

SOCIALISM FOR VETERANS

American politics and culture reject the concept of socialistic government, yet Congress established a socialistic healthcare delivery system for veterans. Using the definition provided by the *Merriam-Webster Dictionary*, notice how the VA health system meets the requirement of government owning and administering a means of production. The Federal government owns and operates the numerous VA hospitals and healthcare facilities throughout the country, and VA staff are government employees. News media regularly reports the complaints of veterans and VA employees of the poor care provided and general mismanagement of the VA services. Veterans enroll on long wait lists to receive services, and once their turn arrives, receive incomplete and otherwise substandard care. If you are not ashamed of how the Federal government consistently fails to meet the healthcare needs of veterans, why aren't you? When considering the VA healthcare system, there is not much to be proud of.

VA HEALTHCARE INEFFICIENCY

The VA system displays incredible inefficiency, and the wait lists for services is only the beginning. The following describes an actual situation I encountered as a home health RN:

The veteran was recently discharged from a local VA hospital, with instructions that the home health nurse would obtain weekly blood specimens for the ordered labs and deliver them to the nearest VA laboratory. The veteran lives about two miles from the closest commercial medical lab, but the nearest VA laboratory to his home is about 15 miles away. Instead of driving about two miles to drop of the lab specimens, I must drive about 15 miles instead, which, of course, means extra paid time and mileage for delivery of the specimens to the VA. I must use lab tubes provided by the VA, as VA labs will not accept the commonly available blood specimen tubes used by most commercial labs, incurring the additional expense of using distinct blood tubes required by the VA.

I draw the blood and drive the specimens the 15 miles to the nearest VA facility. Upon my arrival at the VA lab, the lab tech informs me there "is no order for the labs," even though I produce the copy of the signed discharge instructions from the local VA hospital which clearly states the order for the weekly labs. The lab tech at the VA is not willing to make any effort to correct the discrepancy. I leave the specimens at the reception desk of the VA lab and call the VA physician's office (in the same building as the lab) and inform that team about the specimens delivered to the lab, and the need to resolve the "order" problem if they want results. Otherwise, the blood will not be tested, and the physician will not receive any results.

Approximately two hours later, the VA physician's nurse practitioner calls me reporting resolution of the order problem and the blood has been tested. Let us review all the inefficiencies, unnecessary and avoidable expenses involved with something as simple as drawing a blood sample and dropping it off at a lab:

1. Special blood tubes are required which are only available from the VA.
2. The drive time delivering the specimens about 15 miles, instead of about two miles.
3. Time wasted at the VA lab reception desk trying to convince a lab technician that the written order I could and did produce was indeed an order.
4. The VA lab tech's indifference to the need to confirm the orders. The VA lab tech very clearly communicated how it was my responsibility, a person who is not a VA employee, to resolve the order discrepancy.
5. Extra time wasted calling the VA physician office and talking to the nurse practitioner when she called back.
6. The nurse practitioner wasting time listening to my message, investigating, and resolving the order discrepancy and returning my call.

Consider how that story is only a minor one compared to the numerous barriers veterans encounter every single day at the many VA healthcare facilities throughout the United States. Another example:

Veterans receiving radiation treatment for cancer must be transported for two hours one-way to receive those treatments as their local VA hospital does not provide radiation treatments. The VA provides a daily bus service between the two hospitals. The veteran needing the radiation must arrive at the local VA hospital by 6AM, otherwise the bus departs without him. If he misses the bus, he either misses the radiation treatment or he finds his own transportation for the 4-hour round trip.

He makes the bus, but he must be awake by 4:30AM to be dressed and arrive by 6AM at the local VA hospital. The bus line does not return until all the veterans on the bus complete their appointments at the distant VA hospital. Even though his radiation treatment takes about 15 minutes, he remains at the distant VA hospital until the bus returns the veterans to the local VA hospital. The returning bus often does not return to the local VA hospital until 6PM. By the time he gets home, it is nearly 7PM. Not counting his time preparing and commuting to and from the local VA hospital, he spends 12 hours each day receiving one 15-minute radiation treatment. And he does that Monday through Friday for six weeks of a complete radiation treatment series.

No medical care is available on the bus as the bus service is strictly transportation only. When he becomes ill and vomits on the bus from the radiation treatments, he is on his own, or relies on the other veterans, who are also ill, to assist him. Again, he does that five days per week for six weeks.

Aren't you outraged that ill and injured veterans must endure such wastefulness, discomfort, and humiliation just to receive a medical service? If you are not outraged, why not? If you are not already outraged, consider how the VA has a prioritization process for veterans needing VA medical services. It is not a simple process of enrolling and scheduling appointments and care. In addition to a veteran's income, the location of their residence also affects when their ability to enroll and access VA medical services.

VA PRIORITIZATION

The VA uses all these factors to determine when a veteran will be enrolled with VA healthcare services:

1. The veteran's military service record.
2. Any service-related disability.
3. The veteran's income in relationship to income limits, which are geographically adjusted.
4. Eligibility for Medicaid in the state in which the veteran resides.
5. Veteran eligibility for other benefits such as a VA pension.
6. Veteran willingness to pay copays for services.

The details of the VA prioritization process can be found at this url: https://www.va.gov/health-care/eligibility/priority-groups/. The priority groups range from 1 (soonest) to 8 (latest). Here are some highlights that stood out for me:

- Former POWs and Purple Heart recipients qualify for a Priority Group 3 unless they were awarded a Medal of Honor or a significant service-related disability.
- A "catastrophically disabled" veteran qualifies for Priority Group 4 unless there is another factor that can qualify them for a higher priority.
- Veterans exposed to ionizing radiation from atmospheric testing or during the occupation of the Japanese cities of Hiroshima or Nagasaki qualify for Priority Group 6 unless they qualify for a higher priority.

Hopefully, the thought "Really?" races through your mind as you read each of the three prioritization examples, because that certainly went through my mind. A former POW must wait for medical care from the VA? Really? A catastrophically disabled veteran must wait for medical care from the VA? Really? Veterans exposed to radiation from nuclear weapons must wait for medical care from the VA? Really?

In addition, the "geographically adjusted income limit" results in veterans of lower income in rural areas and states waiting longer than veterans in lower income brackets in more urbanized areas and states. The cost of living in Los Angeles and New York City is significantly higher than in Lincoln, Nebraska or Mansfield, Ohio. Therefore, veterans living in expensive cities qualify to be seen sooner in a VA health facility than those veterans living in rural areas, which reinforces the disparity inherent to the location of most VA hospitals. Most large VA facilities are in large cities which allows veterans residing in and near those metropolitan areas easier transportation to those facilities and more access to services than rural veterans who must travel greater distances.

MEDICARE FOR ALL VETERANS

Now I explain how Medicare For All positively impacts the lives and medical care for all American veterans. And I also describe a reconfiguration of VA healthcare that accommodates Medicare For All.

VETERANS ENROLLED FIRST

Once Congress gains the pollical courage and enacts Medicare For All, implementation needs to be a progressive process because enrolling hundreds of millions of Americans will be an enormous undertaking requiring years of effort. Therefore, I propose veterans and active American military service members enjoy priority and enroll with Medicare For All first, then other population groups will enroll based on a progressive prioritization. Additionally, I propose Congress implement a Medicare secondary payer plan only for veterans and their dependent family members as Congress has already partially provided a secondary payer via the Tricare healthcare coverage for uniformed service members, military retirees, and their families.

RESTRUCTURING VA HEALTHCARE

Currently, veterans covered by both Medicare and VA have the choice of receiving services either separately from Medicare and VA or simultaneously from both. Two major problems exist with that arrangement. First, American taxpayers pay twice to cover the same veteran. Taxpayers pay first via the Medicare payroll tax to cover the veteran, then pay again via other federal taxes for the VA healthcare services. Plus, the two systems poorly communicate with each other. No method of direct communication exists between VA physicians and community physicians billing for Medicare services. I fully endorse American taxpayers having responsibility for paying for 100% of healthcare services for veterans, but I also fully endorse that taxpayers should only pay once to provide that 100% coverage. Hence, my following proposals for restructuring VA healthcare.

MEDICARE IS PRIMARY AND TRICARE IS SUPPLEMENTAL.

Once a veteran enrolls with Medicare For All, that includes automatic enrollment with Tricare as the supplemental health insurance. Medicare with Tricare would then supersede any other health insurance plans such as state Medicaid coverage, employer health insurance or other private health insurance. I also propose that Medicare with Tricare supersede other health insurance coverage such as workers compensation or automobile insurance. Note, there would not be changes to any other benefits under workers compensation or automobile insurance. Imagine the appeal of a veteran candidate to a prospective employer with the employer knowing that the job candidate comes with complete health insurance coverage at no additional expense to the employer! Imagine how much a premium discount could be offered to veterans for automobile insurance with the insurance company not being responsible for covering any acute medical expenses for a veteran injured in an automobile collision! There are numerous wins with a system that fully reimburses Medicare-covered care for veterans: lower automobile premiums for veterans, better access to care regardless of location, no direct employer cost for healthcare benefits for veterans they employ, and complete elimination of the nonsensical enrollment prioritization for the VA.

VA HOSPITALS BILL MEDICARE AND TRICARE

Instead of being separately funded with tax dollars, all VA hospitals and other medical providers would begin billing Medicare and Tricare for services provided to veterans. Medicare regulations and law requires that hospitals that bill Medicare be accredited by The Joint Commission. However, the VA already requires that most of its facilities and providers be Joint Commission accredited. There would be a transition where VA staff and providers implement Medicare and Tricare billing. But there are plenty of consultants and billing agencies already providing such services for current Medicare providers that would be available to either provide that service for the VA or assist the VA with implementing its' own billing system. It is win, win, win and win!

TRANSITIONING VA FACILITIES

Next, the VA transitions VA hospitals and facilities operations to proprietary and nonprofit healthcare providers. As mentioned, the current VA healthcare system is a socialist-style operation with numerous care quality problems. Congress would then authorize for the VA to schedule VA hospitals and other VA healthcare facilities to either be sold or leased to bidding healthcare providers. The winning healthcare corporations would be required to maintain Joint Commission accreditation and assure that all required and current healthcare services to veterans be maintained. Discontinuation or reduction of a service to veterans at a leased or sold VA property would require Congressional approval. Congress should consider establishment of local veteran services boards that would oversee adherence with contracts, quality of care provided and service delivery. The healthcare corporations successfully bidding to operate and/or purchase a VA facility or hospital, would have accountability to the local veteran services board. The local veteran services board would enjoy the authority of approving or disapproving contracts on behalf of Congress. At a minimum, those local veteran services boards would be audited by, and accountable to The House Committee on Veterans Affairs. The local veteran service boards would include veterans residing in the service area of the VA facility, and are an active patient at that VA facility.

The healthcare corporations then bill Medicare and Tricare for services provided. For VA services provided which are not standard Medicare-covered services, such as nursing home care and other long-term-care services, burial, and memorials, et. al., Congress would legislate separately managing those services from Medicare-covered services, avoiding any disruption of the services, benefits, or operations by the VA.

My recommendations to Congress for transitioning current VA healthcare facilities:

1. Create a national VA services oversight board with board members nominated by the President and approved by Congress. Board membership consists of a balance between active and retired military, current VA patients, members of Congress, and members of the Presidential administration. The board reviews, approves, modifies, or denies any applications from regional VA service boards regarding contracts for operations at local VA facilities. Contracts for provision of services at a VA facility are not valid until approved by the national board. Denied applications are appealable to Congress.

2. Create state and/or regional VA services boards with board members nominated by the state governor and approved by the state legislature. Board membership is a balance of active and retired military, current VA patients, state or local representatives and the current gubernatorial administration. All bids and applications from all providers to operate a VA-owned facility would be to the state or regional VA services board. All service provider applications approved by the state or regional VA services board is forwarded to the national VA services board for review and approval. Denied applications may be appealed to the national board.

3. The current Office of the Inspector General of the Department of Veterans Affairs retains all investigation, reporting and oversight of services provided for and to veterans. A Deputy Inspector would be appointed reporting to and advising each state or regional board. The President's authority for removing the Inspector General or a Deputy Inspector is limited to suspension while under investigation. When the President suspends the Inspector General or a Deputy Inspector, the President must immediately notify the House Committee on Veterans Affairs, which then investigates the complaint against the suspended inspector. If the House Committee's investigation finds just cause for removal or other disciplinary action against the accused inspector, following an approved motion by the House, the disciplinary recommendation is forwarded to the United States Senate Committee on Veterans Affairs. If the Senate committee confirms the allegations and recommendations, a majority vote of the Senate confirms and enacts the removal from office or other disciplinary action against the inspector.

TAXPAYERS NOW PAY MORE THAN 100%

An article posted by the *Military Times* website reporting how the VA is responsible for paying for emergency care out-of-pocket expenses for veterans is an excellent example of the ineffective and excessively costly system of healthcare provided by the VA.

Two veterans sued the VA for failure to pay their out-of-pocket expenses when they obtained emergency room care at non-VA facilities. A factor in their decisions to not seek care at a VA hospital was the reality that the closest VA hospital with an ER was several hours drive away, so they went to local hospital ERs instead. The veterans had applied for reimbursement of their out-of-pocket costs that were not covered by health insurance and Medicare. The VA denied the reimbursement applications, and the veterans sued in federal court. The federal court found that the VA had improperly denied the reimbursements and ordered that the VA begin approving and reimbursing those claims for out-of-pocket medical expenses. It is anticipated that the court ruling and subsequent additional reimbursement of out-of-pocket medical expenses for veterans will increase the VA budget by billions of unspecified dollars.

Let's look at all the costs incurred to the American taxpayer in relation to the lawsuit by the two veterans:

1. Medicare coverage for the one veteran already covered by Medicare.
2. Both veterans were already covered by VA healthcare, but could not access emergency services by the VA because of the distance between their residences and the nearest VA hospital ER.
3. The VA hospital and ER that could not be accessed by either veteran.
4. Court costs for operation of the federal court that ruled in favor of the veterans.
5. Legal expenses for the plaintiff veterans.
6. Legal expenses for the VA and federal government to defend against the lawsuit.
7. Reimbursement for out-of-pocket expenses to the two veterans as plaintiffs, and all the other veterans is similar circumstances requiring past, current, and future reimbursement.

Hence, American taxpayers pay for much more than the medical care for the veterans, as they also pay for all the legal costs associated with the lawsuit, and the past, current, and future out-of-pocket expenses for scores of affected veterans.

Now, imagine the costs to the American taxpayer when veterans have coverage under Medicare For All with Tricare as a secondary payer. The costs would be:

1. The initial ER charge for each veteran at the hospital ER of their choice.
2. The copay expense charged to Tricare for the portion of the ER bill not coverage by Medicare.

Americans would pay 100% for the healthcare services to the veterans without all the additional nonmedical legal fees and costs. Plus, the veterans would no longer worry about, or need to know which is the closest VA hospital with an ER—they simply go to the nearest ER and know their medical expenses are covered without future financial headaches for themselves. Such is my vision for honoring all American veterans of our military forces—when they are ill or injured, they obtain the needed medical care as locally as possible, with a minimum of fuss, bother or worry to them about payment. I know I am willing to contribute my tax dollars to their care and comfort, aren't you?

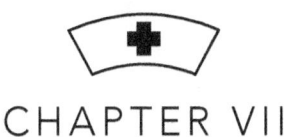

CHAPTER VII

MEDICARE FOR ALL AND CORRECTIONS

MEDICARE FOR ALL AND THE CRIMINAL JUSTICE SYSTEM

Medical care in the nation's jails and prisons has special importance for me as I spent nine years of my nursing career working in prisons. I witnessed firsthand the poor-quality care, excessive costs, and extreme inefficiency. There is one simple explanation for the poor medical care within prisons: correctional administrators suck at managing health care services.

Why are correctional administrators so unable to properly administer medical services? Primarily because the expectation of making decisions for which they lack proper education and preparation and are therefore set up for failure by the competing budget priorities they juggle every day. Licensed healthcare providers such as physicians, registered nurses and nurse practitioners routinely report to an administrative manager without any formal medical education or background. Those licensed medical staffers are then expected to follow the direction of unlicensed persons. If all prison wardens were required to be educated healthcare professionals, that would solve many conflicts with corrections healthcare services. However, wardens and sheriffs and police chiefs maintain the safety and security of the institution and custody of those persons legally incarcerated, and their education and competency are based on those expectations, not the expectation of providing quality healthcare.

The solution resulting in better correctional healthcare services requires divorcing healthcare administration within the institutions from the other administrative duties of wardens and sheriffs and police chiefs. Medicare For All accomplishes that separation, with many benefits. In addition to improving the quality of healthcare within prisons and jails, there would be budget relief for the wardens and sheriffs by eliminating their responsibility for paying for most healthcare services and would relieve them of involvement with medical decision making for inmates and detainees. The quality-of-care improvement would occur because the nurses and physicians and other medical providers would be communicating and collaborating with their licensed peers and would no longer be directly accountable to unlicensed correctional administrators.

An important clarification: Medicare For All coverage for prison and jail populations would only involve those services already covered by Medicare. Routine services provided by correctional institutions such as 24/7 nursing presence would not be covered or included as prisons and jails are residential care facilities, not inpatient facilities, and Medicare already does not cover residential care services, the same a Medicare does not pay for nursing home or assisted living care. Hence, I am advocating for Medicare For All to pay for the same medical products and services as for any other Medicare beneficiary such as prescription medications, physician appointments, labs and medical imaging, outpatient treatments and procedures and inpatient care. Correctional institutions operating as true inpatient facilities would be able to provide and bill Medicare for those inpatient services the same as hospitals and skilled nursing facilities currently bill Medicare.

My ideas for implementing Medicare For All within the criminal justice system:

- All jailed and imprisoned persons who are legal residents of the USA retain their Medicare coverage while incarcerated.

- Wealthy inmates and detainees would remain responsible to pay their portion (20%) of covered medical services. Those inmates and detainees, or their families, could pay the monthly premiums to a private insurance plan for Medicare supplemental insurance.
- Each state or territory creates a Medicaid coverage program for those incarcerated persons covering the 20% of medical charges not covered by Medicare. States and territories would contract with health insurance plans to provide a combined Medicare/Medicaid coverage benefit. Medicare would pay the insurance plan the calculated per-person premium for that state, and the state Medicaid plan would pay the remaining premium and out-of-pocket expenses. Congress would arrange for CMS to provide similar coverage options for persons incarcerated by the Federal Bureau of Prisons.
- Correctional systems through their contracted medical providers would implement system-wide cost-saving systems such as mail-order pharmacies and telehealth.
- Correctional systems contract with Medicare-enrolled healthcare providers and the state Medicaid system for provision and billing of medical services. Consequently, detainees lose the freedom of provider choice, but restriction of providers is essential so that the wardens, sheriffs, and police chiefs assure maintenance of facility safety and security by limiting staff access.

A debatable operational and political problem needing resolution regards managing the health care of persons who are jailed, not yet convicted, and still covered by a Medicare HMO or other MA plan. Each state and territory legislature would arrange reimbursement for healthcare services in jails and prisons with coordination and agreement with CMS. Congress would arrange a reimbursement plan between CMS and for those detained and not-convicted persons in the custody of the Bureau of Prisons.

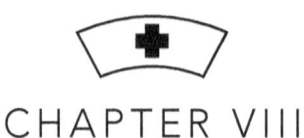

CHAPTER VIII

MEDICARE FOR ALL
AND POLITICS

THE POLITICS OF MEDICARE FOR ALL.

Originally, this book was planned as a strictly empirical and mathematical text, including only facts and the explanations of the taxation formulas that would allow all Americans to finally enjoy universal health care coverage throughout the nation. However, I as researched further, I became increasingly aware of the naivete and futility of ignoring and disregarding the politics of making Medicare For All a reality. Therefore, I include this chapter of my analysis of various arguments for and against Medicare For All.

M4A COULD BE SOCIALISTIC, BUT
IT DOES NOT HAVE TO BE.

Various politicians and pundits complain and warn how Medicare For All would be socialist and lead us to ruination. Socialism is one way to go, as Rand and Kelly Paul, in their book *The Case Against Socialism*, do an excellent job explaining how and why socialism repeatedly fails. I completely agree with the political position that socialism is highly undesirable and would be a completely unworkable and ruinous method for implementation and activation of Medicare For All. But, in her book *Blowout*, Rachel Maddow also superbly explains how capitalist corporations, specifically oil and gas corporations, exploit the evils of socialistic nations and societies and subvert democracy to earn their profits. In addition, oil and gas companies enjoy completely financially unnecessary tax breaks, poison the environment, create unnatural disasters, and receive subsidies for doing so. The energy corporation elites enjoy enormous personal and corporate revenues and profits while endangering the populace and legally avoiding the costs of the many negative impacts of their extraction activities. Proper taxation of polluting industries, such as the oil and gas industry, would even up the score.

The Senator and Ms. Paul provide wonderful examples of the socialistic failures of the USSR, Nazism, and fascism. Although I greatly enjoyed reading *The Case Against Socialism* because of their accurate depiction of the horrific negative consequences of mass murders and profound impoverishment of the lower classes, the senator and his spouse missed a crucial perspective. They did not discuss how American and western capitalism achieves success by collaborating and supporting socialistic governments and societies in other nations. ExxonMobil shares technology and oil and gas extraction profits with Rosneft, the Russian-government-owned oil and gas company. Ms. Maddow documents in detail how Putin created a socialistic successor to the USSR by using the laws and resources of Russian government to eliminate the persons and competitors to the government-owned and operated energy extraction giants. Rosneft and Gazprom are precisely the current examples of socialism that Senator and Ms. Paul revile. I do not recall their mention of Putin being a socialist autocrat or Rex Tillerson, the former U.S. Secretary of State, as the capitalistic enabler of a socialist autocrat.

Likewise, the Pauls fail with explaining or mentioning how the current Trump administration, while professing a distain for socialism, promotes, enables, and defends socialistic autocrats and governments in other countries. The monarchy of Saudi Arabia wages war in Yemen, and then seem completely surprised when their warring opponents figure out how to strike back at the heart of their oil production infrastructure. The Saudi royal family is homophobic, misogynistic and enforces religious discrimination throughout their kingdom, while enforcing complete control over the country's economy and means of production. An excellent example indeed of the despicable socialism described by the Senator and his spouse. Yet, American military forces help defend Saudi Arabia's oil production from their enemies. So much for warning against the horrors of socialism. Socialism is awful for America and Americans but is apparently perfectly acceptable for Saudi and Russian citizens.

Ms. Maddow wonderfully itemizes the evils of unrestrained capitalism, including subjugation of the socially disadvantaged, extensive pollution with environmental destruction and excessive profiteering. It seems the worst of all worlds is how capitalists enjoin with socialists for mutual enabling and support, allowing survival and proliferation of the worst aspects of both economic systems. We need a new path forward.

A DIFFERENT DEFINITION OF SOCIOECONOMICS

Let us review the economic systems, known as economisms, of current and past human history. The economisms are:

1. Capitalism—Private ownership of the means of production.
2. Communism—Communal ownership of the means of production.
3. Feudalism—A monarch controls the means of production.
4. Socialism—Workers, via state-ownership, control the means of production.
5. Statism—Also known as Nazism and fascism, concentrates all power with the state and eliminates personal freedoms.
6. Welfare State—The state assures the economic success and stability of all citizens.

CAPITALISM

Capitalism, the strongest of the economisms, has a dark side. Free markets are the hallmark of capitalism, with individuals permitted unrestricted accumulation of money and property. The acquisitor fulfills as the ideal champion of capitalistic societies. The major strength of capitalism is the strong rewards and incentives for productively and innovations. Consistently throughout American history, those who work hard and create new services and products, thrive. The major weakness of capitalism is its promotion of worsening income equality as elites and wealthy gain ever more wealth while the lower classes struggle meeting daily financial obligations because progressively increasing living expenses consume their lower incomes. Government promotes and reinforces income inequality when the Federal Reserve maintains interest rates so low that lower class citizens with meager savings accounts cannot earn enough interest on their bank accounts to keep up with inflation.

Through the tactic of maintaining interest rates low, the U.S. Federal Reserve reinforces the process of wealth distribution from the middle and lower classes upwards to the wealthy and privileged. By keeping interest rates, and therefore mortgage lending rates low, the already wealthy can more easily afford to purchase real estate, including rental properties and vacation homes. But, the middle and lower classes, who must more carefully budget their money, encounter increased difficulty affording mortgage payments as the excessive realty purchases by the wealthy drive up the values and purchase prices of homes. Lower- and middle-class Americans must pay rent because they cannot afford to purchase a home, and therefore do not gain any equity from their housing. The wealthy continue to gain equity with the rental properties. Real estate becomes over-valued which promotes escalating rents, resulting in a greater percentage of middle- and lower-class incomes being consumed by housing costs.

Another strength of capitalism, integration of an innovation into the economy usually results in a reduction of cost, eventually allowing affordability for all classes of citizens. For example, when Karl Benz first patented the motorcar in 1886, only the wealthy could afford one, the same way wealthier customers can afford purchasing a Tesla automobile today. However, Henry Ford revolutionized industrialization and the automobile industry by refining manufacturing, lowering the cost of production significantly, thereby reducing the purchase price of a Ford automobile. Once the purchase price of a car came within the means of most Americans, Ford's production and success expanded dramatically, eventually replacing the horse and carriage as the primary means of transportation. Ford also paid an improved wage to his employees, which better allowed his employees to become purchasers of Ford automobiles. Note how the purchase price of fully electric vehicles has been decreasing, allowing more people to become purchasers, explaining social class differences as an essential function and component of capitalism. Capitalism needs the wealthy for funding of progress and innovation, but capitalism also promotes progressive cost reduction so that the innovation eventually becomes within the financial means of most citizens. Hence, wealth accumulation is an essential function of the success of capitalism for a nation and society.

However, the great sin of capitalism is also income inequality between social classes. As the wealthy become wealthier, their greater accumulation comes at the expense of the middle and lower classes. Left unchecked, eventually the economy collapses into recessions and depressions because the middle and lower classes have fewer funds for living expenses as those expenses continue to increase while their incomes either decrease or stagnate. Such occurred during the Great Depression of 1929 and the Great Recession of 2009. The wealthy became wealthier by decreasing resources to the lower classes. In 2009, corporations eliminating pension plans and reduced healthcare coverage, improving their bottom lines and therefore their stock performance, which was a contributing mechanism triggering the recession. The company elites, owning much of the company stock, enriched themselves by reducing their employment expenses with lower healthcare and pension costs, which shift to employees. Healthcare cost increases cancel out wage increases. Then, the wealthy drive the stock markets up, using their additional income pulled from the lower classes, until eventually the speculative bubble bursts and the stock market dramatically declines, endangering the financial health of everyone.

The same pattern and process continues. General Motors closes factories and lays off the workers, whose same federal income taxes bailed out General Motors only 10 years ago. Medicare For All would balance the distribution of wealth among the social classes by reducing the financial burden of expensive American healthcare on those who have the least means of affording it.

COMMUNISM

Communist governments control and manage all aspects of commercial and economic activity. Essentially, all citizens of a communist nation are government employees. Although Karl Marx and Friedrich Engels attempted addressing the social and economic disparities of crony capitalism of the Gilded Age, their beliefs and theories possessed a major flaw. They failed accounting for the natural human tendency and need for positive reward for work and effort. Communism does not reward the individual based on personal productivity and expects the individual productivity for the state regardless of level of compensation. Communism also shares a common defect with crony capitalism in that money and resources become concentrated and controlled by the few elite and highly placed government officials while the masses subsist on minimal compensation. Eventually, so many people lose their motivation for productivity that eventually the social and economic activity of the nation collapses because not enough people willingly work at a sufficiently productive level to maintain the economy, and a severe economic depression precedes the collapse of the government. The Soviets were unwilling to make the modifications allowing their nation to survive. In contrast, The People's Republic of China integrates some capitalistic principles, allowing economic growth, lifting hundreds of millions of citizens out of poverty.

FEUDALISM

A "lord" or other master owns and controls the land, and landholders are organized into a hierarchal aristocracy resulting in monarchs and other "royalty" and various lesser titled aristocratic persons and families. The primary means of production is non-mechanized agriculture and most of the populace, called serfs or peasants, are indentured to the master. The master provides protection from attack via knights, soldiers, castles and forts and the profits from the sale and trade of agricultural products returns to the master. Although oil production is the primary commercial activity controlled by royalty, instead of agriculture, Saudi Arabia is a best current example of a persisting feudalistic society. The Saudi royal family controls the economic activity of the entire nation, and all non-royals are obligated to be productive for the sake of the royal family.

SOCIALISM

Free markets may exist somewhat, but government tightly controls primary commercial activity, with large commercial corporations directly owned and operated by the government. The members of government may be "elected," however, government may strictly control and restrict candidacy for offices so that persons elected already support the economic and social dogma of the established government. Socialistic nations encounter a great deal of difficulty managing severe external threats because the rigidity of thought and action suppresses the innovation needed for adaptation to the changing world. As the Pauls point out, socialism usually leads to armed conflict, then the socialist government lacks the financial and social resources to maintain and defend themselves on a long-term basis.

STATISM

The Nazi Third Reich and the Italian fascists lead by Benito Mussolini are excellent examples of the hardship and failure of Statism. Not only does the government control essentially all aspects of commercial enterprise, but Statist regimes also profoundly suppress individual thought, rights, and action. Essentially, individual rights are absent, obligating all citizens to serve the demands and needs of the governmental elites controlling the country. Elections, essentially sham demonstrations of false democracy, consist of candidates pre-selected and pre-approved by the established government as a condition of listing on the ballot. Statist nations becomes utter failures because they both deprive their citizens of the basic resources needed to maintain everyday living while harshly punishing the most minor resistance or disobedience. The general population becomes not only impoverished, but extremely demoralized. Statist nations fail both because they deprive the population of the ability for self and mutual defense, and because the citizenry loses the motivation for resisting external threats.

WELFARE STATE

Welfare states, such as Sweden, provide extensive cradle-to-grave social support programs such as health insurance, paid parental leave and expanded public-funded education. Welfare states exhibit the positive attributes of all citizens sharing the same government program benefits and reduces poverty by assuring the least advantaged have equal access to financial support programs. The primary weakness of welfare states is the requirement for collection of high tax levies. Accumulating wealth in a welfare state nation becomes more difficult because the taxation rates pull revenue away from the wealthy and advantaged and redirects it towards lower social classes via the various government support programs.

Welfare states are stable governments, but commercial progress and innovation slows because resources used by the wealthy to develop new technologies is instead directed towards funding the numerous social support programs. All modern governments must have some means of welfare benefits for their citizens, otherwise, government exists solely for the purpose of satisfying the needs of the elite and wealthy, the primary problem with feudalistic and statist governments. Plus, some social welfare programs provide essential economic compensation and balance when negative economic events occur. For example, the Federal

Deposit Insurance Corporation (FDIC) prevents and manages bank failures by assuring that depositors maintain the value and access to their bank accounts when individual banks fail, and widespread economic downturns occur.

COLLABORISM

I propose the establishment of an updated and progressive economic system of collaborism. Collaborism combines the positive attributes of other economisms with capitalism as the base socioeconomic system. Collaborism retains these positive characteristics of capitalism:

- Private ownership of the means of production. Individuals continue ownership of private and publicly traded companies, however, all employees become "associates" and a portion of labor compensation includes awarding of voting stock, the same as executive leaders and board members of proprietary corporations are similarly compensated. Labor unions would eventually become obsolete because workers integrate into the governing social structure of the company, allowing them input into corporate decision making and promoting joint accountability throughout the corporation. The mutual interests of the workers merge with the corporate interests.

- Free markets with minimal government intervention. The Great Depression and various other severe financial downturns of the 19th, 20th and 21st centuries explain the hazards and undesirability of unrestricted and unregulated free markets. However, government regulation and oversight needs limiting to assuring protection of citizens and consumers in the least restrictive manner possible. Returning to the FDIC example, the FDIC regulates banks, assuring they operate properly, but avoid involvement with assuring individual bank success.

- Promotion of progress, reform, and innovation. An essential factor with all social and technological progress is sufficient financial resources for investment in new ideas and methods.

Tesla automobiles, priced above the range of most American's affordability, must be initially highly priced. Developing the technologies and devices needed for transitioning to a fully electronic vehicle is quite expensive and requires the financial resources that wealthy customers and investors provide. In this manner, the wealthy provide a very essential function to national and societal growth and development. As the technology matures, and especially when applicable patents expire, and competitors more freely engage the market with their own similar products, the price of fully electronic vehicles will continue declining until most citizens can afford that purchase. This process occurs already as other manufactures of fuel-powered vehicles currently develop their own versions of electric powered vehicles.

- Individual liberties and rights remain unchanged. There are no modifications to the Bills of Rights, or any of the other rights established by statutory or common law. Free and fair markets require the participation of free and fair citizens.

Collaborism offers these modifications to capitalism, some of which are already in effect:

- Increased "assigned" taxation. With assigned taxation, the tax collection restricts spending of the funds. Social Security is an excellent example of how this collaborism principle works: Payroll taxes collected for Social Security retirement and disability benefits are used only for payment and administration of Social Security benefits. Congress lacks any discretion with spending those funds on any other purpose. The current Medicare payroll tax already works in this manner as well. That payroll tax exclusively funds administration and payment of Medicare-covered benefits. Another example of assigned taxation is fuel taxes devoted to construction and maintenance of the nation's roadways. Assigned taxation has also been referred to as "earmarked" taxes.

- Better distribution of social supports without direct distribution of revenue to the poor and other disadvantaged persons and groups. One of the valid complaints about welfare programs regards direct payments to recipients creates a financial incentive lessening participation with active work and receipt of personal income from an employer or from self-employment. However, some persons and groups simply cannot contribute to the workplace because of valid disabilities. People with intellectual disabilities often cannot participate in the mainstream workforce but can participate in sheltered workshops where the employer accommodates their specific needs to overcome the barriers to productive work.

- Acceptance of a higher tax burden by the wealthy. Many wealthy persons seek recognition of their charitable donations and efforts. However, it is also generous to pay a greater percentage of taxes both as a means of being charitable to the nation at large and preventing the negative consequences of poverty by funding government programs aimed at poverty abatement. An example could be creating a surtax on highly priced real estate and use of the surtax solely for creation of low-cost housing and other programs reducing homelessness.

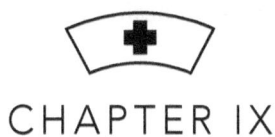

CHAPTER IX

MODERN AMERICAN SLAVERY

MODERN AMERICAN SLAVERY

Unfortunately, prescription American healthcare possesses all the trappings of chattel slavery, an interesting contradiction considering the USA has the 13th Amendment to the Constitution prohibiting slavery, and Americans fought each other during the Civil War defeating slavery.

We now examine how chattel slavery shares common elements with the current "health" care insurance "system" in the United States of America:

- A master/slave dependency.
- Endemic racism.
- A mechanism of economic enforcement.
- Similar risks of injury and death.
- Political and government structures create and reinforces the system.
- Both subjugate large numbers of laborers.
- The primary means of escape is leaving the USA.

Prior to The Emancipation Proclamation in 1863, slaves were economically dependent to their masters. Currently, most workers covered by employer health insurance are also dependent on the employer as health insurance coverage does not transfer between employers. In a paper on racial and ethnic disparities with health insurance coverage, Heeju Sohn at UCLA describes how both African Americans and Hispanics endure the lowest rates of health insurance coverage. Both systems exhibit racism in that most American slaves were African American, and as Ms. Sohn reports, the largest group of persons in America without health insurance are also African American. The Fugitive Slave Act legally enforced chattel slavery as the Anti-Kickback Law and the Stark Law enforce worker dependence on employer insurance. The extremely unsafe working conditions American slaves endured risked their injury and death daily. Being without health insurance, or being underinsured, risks injury and death from the inability to pay for needed preventive care and treatments, services, and medications. The US Congress and the state legislatures created laws establishing and supporting slavery and established and support the current structure for health insurance coverage.

American slaves numbered in the millions prior to their emancipation, and the millions of current American workers easily outnumbers the upper-class owners of corporations dictating the details of employer-provided health care coverage. And finally, especially after passage of the Fugitive Slave Act, the only escape from slavery was to leave the territory of the USA, such as via the Underground Railroad, as non-slave states could no longer harbor escaped slaves from the South. Similarly, the primary means of escaping the current health care insurance system in the USA is emigration.

Everyone wants "health" care, and no one wants to overpay for anything. In the USA, Americans do not have "health" care and vastly overpay for illness-related products and services. This situation is the consequence of many decades of well-intentioned political choices. The plan was provision of care to specific groups as needs arose. The political plan did not have any leaders with the foresight to understand how the patchwork of solutions resulted in the current circumstances.

AMERICAN "HEALTH" CARE PROBLEMS

"Health" is used in quotations, because the "system" of "health" care is actually sickness-care. Few covered services are truly health and illness-prevention oriented. Coverage of vaccines and full coverage of an annual physical are two examples of health care. However, most services sought by consumers and provided by hospitals, physicians and other providers treats illness and injury and the recovery from illness and injury. "System" is also in quotations as America does not truly have a distinct coordinated system of provision of care. In addition to the government plans of Medicare, Medicaid and VA, there are numerous private health insurance companies and third-party administrators for self-insuring employers.

In addition to the multiple payers, there are multiple overlapping providers, and underserved areas. Metropolitan areas share several networks of care providers, while many rural areas experience shortages of physicians and other providers. Those with regular Medicare coverage may travel anywhere in the USA without a loss of coverage. For those covered under an HMO, service areas and providers are restricted, and care access care while traveling could be significantly limited. Veterans may receive services from the VA system, but endure long wait times. Veterans covered by both Medicare and VA often choose receiving some services from VA, and other services via Medicare reimbursement, and both provider networks lack good communication between them.

Waste in "health" care is rampant. People receive medicines they do not want and accumulate stocks of drugs because the number of meds is too difficult for them to manage. And, if enrolled with automatic refills from a mail-order pharmacy, the refills continue arriving regardless of if the person is taking the drug correctly, or at all.

Medicines are often prescribed based upon marketing outreach from pharmaceutical manufacturers, rather than outcome improvement and cost benefit. For example, warfarin, a commonly prescribed anticoagulant (blood thinner) requires regular blood testing to assure correct dosing. Other available anticoagulants have the same blood thinning effect without the blood testing requirement. But the newer anticoagulants are dramatically more expensive. For the newer anticoagulant, a patient could easily encounter a $200-300 copay each month, with insurance coverage. With insurance coverage, generic warfarin is a monthly copay of a few dollars. Including the cost of the blood test, the total out-of-pocket expense for most patients on warfarin is less than $100 per month.

MEDICARE FOR ALL IS EMANCIPATION OF ALL

Having Medicare cover every single American citizen would truly result in emancipation of all American citizens, which is precisely why politicians, social elites, health insurance companies, pharmaceutical manufacturers and others invested in the current dysfunctional system actively work at defeating the idea. Politicians deny equal coverage for all, while they enjoy full health insurance coverage on the taxpayer's dime. The current situation can be accurately described as a "Gilded Age" of health care like the 19th century industrialists who paid low wages, and disregarded workplace safety while they earned extraordinary rewards on the backs of the laborers. Which was precisely how chattel slavery operated, the primary difference being the workers of the Gilded Age were not considered the property of the industrialists.

Let us examine how Medicare for All Americans would affect the similarities between chattel slavery and elements of the current health care system:

MASTER/SLAVE DEPENDENCY

This relationship ends. The master/slave dynamic dies as the American voter becomes the decision-maker. Persons covered by the insurance become the persons making the decisions about coverage as they chose elected the politicians based on mutual health care needs and resources.

ENDEMIC RACISM

Racial and ethnic disparities terminate. Each American has the same basic Medicare coverage as the next, regardless of age, gender, race, ethnicity, sexual orientation or whatever.

MECHANISM OF ECONOMIC ENFORCEMENT

Economic enforcement continues, but in a different manner. To afford the increased cost of coverage for all Americans, the Medicare payroll tax would increase, and the increase includes increased payroll contributions by workers, by employers and taxes on non-wage income such as capital gains and other non-labor-related income.

SIMILAR RISK OF INJURY AND DEATH

Injury and death risks would decline because financial incentives contributing to avoidance of seeking medical care reduces as well. Preventable diseases become more preventable as more Americans seek better primary care services, rather than waiting until a chronic illness becomes severe and unmanageable.

POLITICAL AND GOVERNMENT STRUCTURE CREATES AND REINFORCES THE SYSTEM

Like the change of economic enforcement, politicians become directly accountable to taxpaying voters, encouraging politicians to enact health care legislation that resolves the many problems with the current system.

SUBJUGATION OF LARGE NUMBERS OF LABORERS

The subjugation based on healthcare coverage and access recedes. Social class distinctions related to basic health care coverage for American citizens and legal residents of the USA no longer exist.

THE PRIMARY MEANS OF ESCAPE IS TO LEAVE THE USA

This element would not change much. But, after the other disparities and inequalities of health care coverage become resolved, a motive to emigrate no longer includes the absence of sufficient health care coverage.

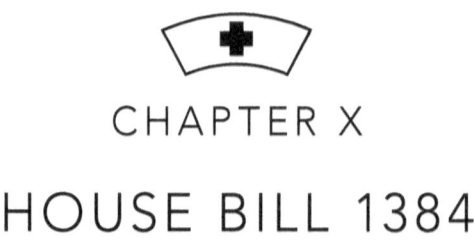

CHAPTER X

HOUSE BILL 1384

H.B. 1384

During the first session of the 116th Congress, Representative Pramila Jayapal of the 7th congressional district of the State of Washington, introduced the "Medicare For All Act of 2019." Although I also list this bill in the references, I include also this link for viewing and downloading the text of the bill: https://www.congress.gov/116/bills/hr1384/BILLS-116hr1384ih.pdf. Here is my list of the flaws with the proposed legislation:

1. Title I, Sec. 102, Universal Coverage specifies the Secretary of Health and Human Services (HHS) shall create a rule specifying defining who is a resident of the United States of America qualifying for coverage under the Medicare benefit. This provision simply allows Congressional avoidance of responsibility for defining who is and who is not a legal resident of the country. Plus, it would permit changing the definition by subsequent HHS Secretaries as political winds blow between successive presidential administrations. Congress should own its responsibility to American citizens by defining those eligible for coverage in the text of the bill and eliminate the option of political gamesmanship.

2. Title I, Sec. 106. (a), requires benefits be established within two years of passage of the bill. Considering that enrollment would involve hundreds of millions of Americans, I am very skeptical that the Social Security Administration and the Centers for Medicare and Medicaid Services possesses the administrative capacity to meet that deadline. If those agencies can meet that deadline, both agencies should explain how they can meet the deadline before the deadline is imposed. I suggest this timeline and deadlines for enrollment:

   a. All veterans, active military and their families, and all newborns enroll within one year of passage.
   b. All children up to age 18, not enrolled as newborns enrolled within 2 years of passage.
   c. All adults aged 50 to 65 years enrolled within 3 years.
   d. All adults aged 35 to 50 years enrolled within 4 years.
   e. All other adults enroll within 5 years of passage.

3. Title I, Sec.107 prohibits duplication of coverage by any private health insurer or any employer. Why would we do that? In a separate chapter, I explain the value of maintain the relationship between private health insurance plans and Medicare via Medicare Advantage and I reiterate the lack of wisdom or value with outlawing private health insurance. Plus, since states, counties, townships, and municipalities are employers, I suspect this provision would violate a state right to manage their own intrastate commerce. If private insurance and states create better health insurance plans competing with Medicare coverage, I cannot think of any reasonable purpose for outlawing it. In addition, persons legally present in the U.S.A., but not residents, such as tourists and visa holders would still need private insurance plans to provide health insurance coverage while they are present in America.

4. Title II, Sec. 201 (a)(7) specifies the coverage of "comprehensive reproductive, maternity and newborn care." I have no argument against, and I greatly encourage the coverage of maternity and

newborn care. However, I suspect "comprehensive reproductive care" includes services such as nontherapeutic abortions, condoms, birth control pills and devices and "morning after" medications. Hopefully, the vagueness of the statement "comprehensive reproductive care" combined with the current state of abortion politics in America, leads one to realize how that provision is a poison pill that many Americans and American politicians are not going to swallow.

5. Title II, Sec. 201 (a)(13) adds the benefit of medical appointment transportation for the disabled and those with low incomes. I object to the addition of an expensive benefit to Medicare coverage. Disabled and low-income Americans already may obtain transportation assistance to medical appointments via the state Medicaid programs. I am not seeing a good reason to change that current arrangement.

6. Title II, Sec. 201 (d) allows the HHS Secretary to include complimentary and integrative medicine practices as a covered Medicare benefit. Again, this provision increases the Medicare benefit to coverage of items and services not currently covered. Congress should negotiate with proponents of coverage of such services and products and not delegate it to a political appointee that changes during and with each successive presidential administration.

7. Title II, Sec. 202 eliminates all out-of-pocket expenses by eliminating all cost-sharing. Please recognize this provision for the bribe that it is. This provision would dramatically increase the cost of healthcare expenses by Medicare by eliminating the current annual deductibles, copays, and co-insurance. All health care decisions involve a consumer purchase. Eliminating out-of-pocket expenses for consumers removes the motive for any American to thoughtfully consider the financial impact of any medical decision. Cost-sharing discourages abuse and fraud and encourages thoughtful discussion and decision making between patients, families, and physicians.

8. Title II, Sec. 204 adds coverage of long-term services to the Medicare benefit. As with the cost-sharing elimination, complementary and integrative services and medical transportation benefit, this provision significantly increases Medicare coverage, and therefore the cost as state Medicaid programs already cover long-term services for disabled and low-income residents. The provision also permits the HHS Secretary wide discretion determining what long-term services shall be covered. As with the other provisions that would increase the Medicare benefit, providers of long-term services should negotiate with Congress for coverage, and not with a political appointee.

9. Title VIII, Sec. 522 (b) requires workers compensation programs reimburse Medicare for medical expenses for work-related injuries. I dislike this concept because it places the injured worker between the federal government and state worker compensation programs whenever a dispute regarding which services workers compensation covers. If Medicare becomes the primary payer for all healthcare in the USA, regardless of origin of the illness or injury, such disputes are eliminated. Workers can receive the needed medical care for recovery from work-related injuries without the stress and worry of having to argue with state and federal bureaucrats and eliminates healthcare provider involvement in such disputes. Adjusting worker compensation programs costs and premiums downward, compensating for the medical services now covered by Medicare would resolve the issue. States would continue providing coverage of cost sharing expenses for the injured worker.

10. Title IX, Sec. 903 terminates the pay for performance programs. What an incredibly bad idea. CMS has been working for many years to implement pay for performance, known as P4P or value-based purchasing. P4P is a major step forward for reimbursement of healthcare services by Medicare. Essentially, providers having the best outcomes for their patients are paid a bonus for the

higher quality of care. Conversely, poorly performing providers receive less reimbursement due to their poor outcomes. The money taken from the poor performers pays the bonuses to the good performers. It is an excellent application of the principles of capitalism. Under P4P, healthcare providers compete for customers and market share, and compete for quality of care. P4P is not only a good thing, but also an exceptionally good thing that has been long overdue, and very capitalistic.

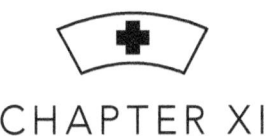

CHAPTER XI

IMPLEMENTING MEDICARE FOR ALL

IMPLEMENTATION

Implementation of M4A requires coordination of two processes—implementing the taxes funding M4A and implementing coverage for all Americans. The Centers for Medicare and Medicaid Services (CMS) and the Social Security Administration would both require progressive implementation of both processes, therefore minimizing disruption of government functioning, economic adjustment, and healthcare operations.

Fully implementing the proposed tax structure quickly would likely result in significant economic disruption because initially taxpayers and employers and producers would pay both the full tax, and the current healthcare premiums, which would be simply unaffordable. Therefore, taxes would increase in a stair-step manner as additional Americans enroll with Medicare and employers and reduce their healthcare insurance premiums offsetting the cost of the tax increases.

In addition, attempting to enroll hundreds of millions of Americans with Medicare For All, including enrollment with Medicare MA plan options would simply overwhelm the current capabilities of any government agency. Congress must prioritize which citizens enroll so enrollment and payment of claims can be processed with minimal delays.

TAX IMPLEMENTATION

For the payroll tax increase, I propose a 0.5% increase each year for both the employee and employer, over a four-year period. For the fifth year of implementation, the payroll tax would increase by 0.55% for both employee and employer, which would then achieve the full 8% payroll deduction tax. Keep in mind, currently 2.9% total payroll tax for Medicare is already paid between the employee and employer. Hence, the payroll tax is increasing by a total of 5.1% to reach the 8% rate. The stair-step tax structure would look like this:

	PXw	+	PXe	=	PX
Current	1.45	+	1.45	=	2.9
Year 1	1.95	+	1.95	=	3.9
Year 2	2.45	+	2.45	=	4.9
Year 3	2.95	+	2.95	=	5.9
Year 4	3.45	+	3.45	=	6.9
Year 5	4	+	4	=	8

For the toxin and other taxes, I propose that 50% of each tax rate be collected for the first two years of implementation, then the remainder tax rate collected in full thereafter.

ENROLLMENT IMPLEMENTATION

I recommend distributing enrollment of citizens over a five-year period with this sequence:

1. Year one and thereafter-All newborns upon birth (registration with the SSA for assignment of a Social Security number), and all veterans and spouses and all active military and their families.

2. Year two and thereafter-All children up to age 18 not already enrolled as a newborn. All children covered by SCHIP (State Children Health Insurance Plan) state Medicaid plans would be enrolled before children not covered by a SCHIP plan. Children born within the territory of the USA are citizens, so native-born American children would be enrolled regardless of the immigration status of their parents. Children illegally within the USA would not be eligible for enrollment or coverage as any other person illegally present in the USA. A new newborn is eligible for enrollment upon birth within the USA, regardless of the immigration status of the mother.

3. Year three and thereafter-All adults aged 50 to 65 not already enrolled.

4. Year four and thereafter—All adults aged 35 to 50 not already enrolled.

5. Year Five and thereafter—All remaining adults not already enrolled.

The U.S. Census Bureau estimates on July 1, 2018, the total population of the USA was 327,167,434. Assuming continued population growth, and simplifying the calculation, I round the American population up to 330 million residents. And CMS reports that 60 million Americans were enrolled as Medicare beneficiaries in 2018, leaving 270 million Americans remaining to be enrolled with Medicare For All. Assuming the five-year implementation plan is adopted, 54 million Americans (270/5 = 54) would be enrolled with Medicare For All each year of implementation. And yes, that means the Social Security Administration would be remarkably busy enrolling citizens with Medicare For All as 4.5 million Americans would need to be newly enrolled each month (54 million per year/12months = 4.5). However, once full enrollment has been achieved, time and cost for enrollment would decline significantly as thereafter, the only enrollments with Medicare would be for newborns and newly legal immigrants. Plus, enrollment would not require application and would become automatic. The Social Security Administration would issue a Medicare card when the person became eligible.

Another detail of enrolling every American is the effective date of enrollment. Currently, enrolling in Medicare, assuming no errors, results in coverage on the first day of the month following enrollment. So, a citizen enrolled on February 15th, has an effective coverage date of March 1st. At a minimum, that effective date process would be retained. However, due to the volume of enrollment that the Social Security Administration and the Centers for Medicare and Medicaid Services would encounter, Congress may wish to create a process extending the time between enrollment and coverage. An extension of the enrollment-to-coverage time may also be required for private insurance plans to properly enlist those newly covered persons with a Medicare Advantage plan.

A potential complication could be enrollment of newborns upon birth, especially if the newborn has a birth complication requiring expensive hospitalization and medical intervention. Obviously, waiting until the first of the month following the birth of the infant is not going to work. Plus, I think an effective incentive to reduce elective abortions is assuring coverage of the fetus throughout pregnancy so that Medicare coverage is active during labor and delivery. Two potential solutions would be for either a method for coverage of the newborn under the mother's Medicare number until the Medicare number for the newborn can be created by Social Security, or creation of the Medicare number for the fetus while in-utero. The fetus of a mother illegally present in the USA would not be covered while in-utero.

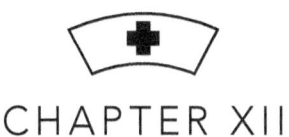

CHAPTER XII

TAKE AWAYS AND NEXT STEPS

TAKE-AWAYS AND NEXT STEPS

After reading my proposals, concepts, and ideas for Medicare For All, I hope you agree with these take-aways:

1. Regardless if Congress fails enacting a Medicare For All law, healthcare services will persistently consume almost 18% of the gross national product. The equation I offer allows all Americans the benefits of better coverage, reduced waste, and better cost control.
2. American veterans suffer a lousy deal. They endure a socialistic healthcare provider system that fails at meeting their needs, does not consistently or reliably provide healthcare services to all veterans and wastes tax dollars and other resources.
3. American taxpayers deserve a better deal towards for tax dollars spent providing healthcare to veterans. Medicare For All combined with Tricare for all veterans would provide better coverage, more accessible services and reduce large amounts of wasted tax dollars and government resources. Additionally, Medicare For All plus Tricare provides a financial incentive for employers to offer jobs to veterans.

4. The current system of healthcare insurance in the USA subsidizes large profitable corporations producing toxic and injurious chemical substances without bearing the true cost of the injury and illness those chemicals and substances inflict. Industries producing harmful substances spawning illness and injury should contribute a fairer share towards the medical costs of treating those injuries and illnesses.

5. Medicare For All takes a huge step towards true equality for all Americans because all American citizens and legal residents of the USA would share the same minimum healthcare insurance coverage. The current divisions of healthcare coverage linked to race, ethnicity and social class see dramatic reductions.

6. Americans have a long tradition and history of supporting and assisting one another. Once again, all Americans can individually and jointly make the changes and sacrifices needed to provide for a better future for each and all of us. As the Founding Fathers committed us with the ratification of the Constitution, Medicare For All is an opportunity to, "…promote the general welfare and secure the blessings of liberty to ourselves and our posterity."

7. Wealthy Americans may choose being more shareful. Medicare For All should not impoverish anyone, and should enrich all Americans with a minimal, reliable healthcare benefit. The wealthy benefit from Medicare For All because they too would have the same minimal healthcare coverage, and because the business expense of providing healthcare insurance for employees would become more consistent and manageable, improving the bottom lines of corporate financial statements.

8. Success with Medicare For All requires every American adult embrace holding the government accountable for wise use of tax dollars. That means making political decisions and voting choices based on results and good ideas instead of fears, bigotry and judgementalism.

NEXT STEPS

It would seem obvious how the next step towards implementing M4A would be for the US Congress to enact the legislation establishing Medicare coverage for all Americans, including approving the tax increases necessary for proper funding of the benefits. If only it were that easy. In addition to Congress legislating the expansion of Medicare, the law would need to be crafted in such a manner to avoid any legal pitfalls that could allow the federal courts to invalidate the law. And, the US President must also sign the law, or Congress must generate sufficient votes overriding a presidential veto.

As complicated as that all sounds, the next step is you. Yes, you. M4A will not happen until most American voters demand Congress act, and the President approves. Although American democracy is incredibly messy, it is also quite effective, and The Constitution of The United States of America functions and operates precisely as the Founding Fathers intended.

The reality of American politics, since gaining independence and the founding of the nation, is Americans excel at uniting when defeating a common threat, then once neutralizing the threat, revert to our argumentative, disagreeable selves. Such has been the circumstances of our democracy since colonial times. The colonists disagreed greatly among themselves, and many of the colonies had border disputes between them. Vermont declared independence as a republic and separated from New Hampshire, which also involved land and boundaries disagreements with New York. While both still colonies, New York and New Jersey disputed their common boundary. And the Mason Dixon Line was surveyed to resolve border disputes between Pennsylvania, Maryland, and Delaware.

The COVID-19 pandemic threatens everyone. Anyone can become ill and die from it. Anyone can transmit the disease to friends, family, acquaintances, coworkers, and strangers. Record-breaking unemployment threatens the safety and security of the unemployed most directly, but also threatens the safety and security of the remaining employed as the national debt escalates, and the financial health of local medical providers deteriorates. The increase of unemployed will result in an increase in the uninsured inability to pay medical bills. Even though many of the unemployed may qualify for financial assistance with health insurance premiums, many will not qualify for any assistance. Hospitals, especially rural hospitals serving areas without any other inpatient provider, will struggle more to meet expenses on lowered revenues. Retail stores are not required to provide services to anyone regardless of ability to pay, but hospitals are required, and do provide regardless of ability to pay.

We share a common threat affecting every American, making it time for all Americans to unite to defeat the threat both medically and economically, and Medicare For All is the response that will defeat the threats from COVID-19.

The Founding Fathers got the Constitution right, in that the Constitution provides precisely as it was intended, by establishing a method for government of the people, for the people and by the people. But the people must demand elected politicians make the changes necessary for our own protection and security, which begins at the ballot box.

Hence, the next step to achieve Medicare For All is for most American voters to choose their representatives and government officers in state and federal positions based upon their willingness to negotiate and establish the federal and state laws needed to fully implement M4A.

The U.S. House of Representatives and the U.S. Senate both need a majority of elected members enacting a Medicare For All law. Each of the state and territorial legislatures requires a majority of elected members creating the supporting legislation that will provide for coverage of the 20% of healthcare services excluded from Medicare reimbursement. We need a President supporting and signing a Medicare For All law, and we need state governors supporting and signing legislation enabling coverage for the remaining 20% of coverage.

The time is now for all Americans to live up to the promises of the Constitution of forming a more perfect union, establishing justice, ensuring domestic tranquility, provide for our common defense, promote our general welfare and secure the blessing of liberty for ourselves and our posterity.

REFERENCES

FACT CHECKING

In the worlds of journalism and internet search, fact-checking is an essential element of information transparency. Without fact-checking, how would anyone know with certainty what is truthful and what is not? In the academic world, fact-checking is known as references. Therefore, I provide references, so all readers know with certainty the math of Medicare For All is based on real numbers from reliable sources. Feel free to do your own fact checking. I specifically sought out references readily available on the internet, and from sources with a reputation for objectivity and reliability. Where a political opinion is stated, that is the opinion of that author, or as reported by that author, and not necessarily the opinion of this author.

If an error, inconsistency or needed refinement is discovered, please post a reply at my blog site, https://nursebarry.com/. Political-opinion-only replies will not garner my attention. However, responding with updated or corrected facts and figures is of great interest to me. When posting a reply, please include any references, calculations, or other facts supporting the response.

REFERENCES

Bureau of Labor Statistics. March 31, 2020. May 2019 National Occupational Employment and Wage Estimates United States. U.S. Department of Labor. Washington D.C. Retrieved from: https://www.bls.gov/oes/current/oes_nat.htm#00-0000.

Bureau of Labor Statistics. September 17, 2019. News Release: Employer Costs for Employee Compensation-June 2019. USDL-19-1649. U.S. Department of Labor. Washington D.C. Retrieved from: https://www.bls.gov/news.release/pdf/ecec.pdf.

Burningham, G. November 4, 2019. The price of insulin has soared. These biohackers have a plan to fix it. *Time*, pp. 74-79. Time USA, LLC. New York, NY.

Case, A. & Deaton, A. March 2-9, 2020. The Sickness of Our System; health care costs undermine working-class lives. *Time*. Time USA, LLC. New York, NY.

Centers for Disease Control and Prevention. July 23, 2019. Economic Trends in Tobacco. U.S. Department of Health and Human Services. Atlanta, GA. Retrieved from: https://www.cdc.gov/tobacco/data_statistics/fact_sheets/economics/econ_facts/index.htm.

Centers for Medicare and Medicaid Services. December 4, 2019. CMS Fast Facts. U.S. Department of Health and Human Services. Baltimore, MD. Retrieved from: https://www.cms.gov/Research-Statistics-Data-and-Systems/Statistics-Trends-and-Reports/CMS-Fast-Facts.

Centers for Medicare and Medicaid Services. n.d. How hospice works. U.S. Department of Health and Human Services. Baltimore, MD. https://www.medicare.gov/what-medicare-covers/what-part-a-covers/how-hospice-works.

Centers for Medicare and Medicaid Services. December 05, 2019. NHE fact sheet. U.S. Department of Health and Human Services. Baltimore, MD. Retrieved from: https://

www.cms.gov/research-statistics-data-and-systems/
statistics-trends-and-reports/nationalhealthexpenddata/
nhe-fact-sheet.

Centers for Medicare and Medicaid Services, Office of the Actuary, National Health Statistics Group. n.d. The Nation's Healthcare Dollar ($3.5 Trillion), Calendar Year 2017, Where It Came From, and The Nation's Healthcare Dollar ($3.5 Trillion), Calendar Year 2017, Where It Went. U.S. Department of Health and Human Services. Baltimore, MD. Retrieved from: https://www.cms.gov/Research-Statistics-Data-and-Systems/ Statistics-Trends-and-Reports/NationalHealthExpendData/ Downloads/PieChartSourcesExpenditures.pdf.

Centers for Medicare and Medicaid Services. n.d. HHS FY 2017 Budget in Brief – CMS -Medicare. U.S. Department of Health and Human Services. Baltimore, MD. Retrieved from: https://www. hhs.gov/about/budget/fy2017/budget-in-brief/cms/medicare/ index.html#parts.

Congressional Budget Office. May 2019. Key Design Components and Considerations for Establishing a Single-Payer Health Care System. Congress of the United States. Washington D.C. Retrieved from: https://www.cbo.gov/system/files/2019-05/55150-singlepayer.pdf.

Conway, J. August 9, 2019. Total Alcohol Beverage Sales in the U.S. 2006-2018. Statista. New York, NY. Retrieved from: https:// www.statista.com/statistics/207936/us-total-alcoholic-beverage s-sales-since-1990/.

Countryeconomy.com. n.d. United States (USA) GDP -Gross Domestic Product. Retrieved from: https://countryeconomy.com/gdp/ usa?year=2017.

Crowell & Moring. January 15, 2003. Ohio Supreme Court Grants $32.5 Million Punitive Damages in Challenge to Benefit Denial and Review Process. Washington, D.C. Retrieved from: https://

www.crowell.com/NewsEvents/AlertsNewsletters/all/Ohi
o-Supreme-Court-Grants-325-Million-Punitive-Damages-in-
Challenge-to-Benefit-Denial-and-Review-Process.

Denison, R. April 14, 2014. Report: Staggering amounts of toxic
chemicals produced across America. Environmental Defense
Fund. New York, NY. Retrieved from: https://www.edf.
org/blog/2014/04/14/report-staggering-amounts-toxi
c-chemicals-produced-across-america.

Department of Veterans Affairs. October 15, 2019. VA Priority Groups.
Washington D.C. Retrieved from: https://www.va.gov/
health-care/eligibility/priority-groups/.

Department of Veterans Affairs. May 9, 2017. Accreditation of Medical
Facilities and Ambulatory Programs; VA Directive 1100.16;
Transmittal Sheet. Washington, D.C. Retrieved from: https://
www.va.gov/vhapublications/ViewPublication.asp?pub_
ID=5396.

Federal Motor Carrier Safety Administration; U.S. Department of
Transportation. August 2018. 2018 Pocket Guide to Large
Truck and Bus Statistics. Washington, D.C. Retrieved from:
https://www.fmcsa.dot.gov/sites/fmcsa.dot.gov/files/docs/
safety/data-and-statistics/413361/fmcsa-pocket-guide-201
8-final-508-compliant-1.pdf.

Federal Trade Commission. 2019. Cigarette Report for 2017.
Washington, D.C. Retrieved from: https://www.ftc.gov/
system/files/documents/reports/federal-trade-commission-ciga
rette-report-2017-federal-trade-commission-smokeless-tobacco-
report/ftc_cigarette_report_2017.pdf.

Federal Trade Commission. 2019. Smokeless Tobacco Report for
2017. Washington, D.C. Retrieved from: https://www.ftc.gov/
system/files/documents/reports/federal-trade-commission-ciga
rette-report-2017-federal-trade-commission-smokeless-tobacco-
report/ftc_smokeless_tobacco_report_2017.pdf.

Government of Canada. July 11, 2017. Health Care in Canada. Canada's Universal Health-care System. Gouvernement du Canada. Ottawa, ON. Retrieved from: https://www.canada.ca/en/ immigration-refugees-citizenship/services/new-immigrants/ new-life-canada/health-care-card.html.

Jacques, J., ND. Winter 2008. A Not-So-Sweet-Story – High Fructose Corn Syrup. Obesity Action Coalition. Tampa FL. Retrieved from: https://4617c1smqldcqsat27z78x17-wpengine.netdna-ssl. com/wp-content/uploads/HFCS.pdf.

Jayapal, P., et. al. February 27, 2019. H.R. 1384. A Bill. To establish an improved Medicare for All national health insurance program. United States House of Representatives. 116th Congress, 1st Session. Washington D.C. Retrieved from: https://www. congress.gov/116/bills/hr1384/BILLS-116hr1384ih.pdf.

Kahn, J.; Sachs, J.; Fremstad, A. et. al. February 28, 2020. Economists conclude that Medicare for All (M4A) could be considerably less expensive than the current healthcare finance system. The Hopbrook Institute. Amherst, MA. Retrieved from: https://www. hopbrook-institute.org/single-post/2020/02/28/Economist s-conclude-that-Medicare-for-All-M4A-could-be-consider ably-less-expensive-than-the-current-healthcare-finance-system.

King, BA; Gammon, DG; Marynak KL; Rogers T. Electronic Cigarette Sales in the United States, 2013-2017. *JAMA*. 2018;320(13):1379– 1380. doi:10.1001/jama.2018.10488. Retrieved from: https:// jamanetwork.com/journals/jama/fullarticle/2705175.

Klurfeld, D.M.; Foreyt, J.; Angelopoulos, T.J. and Rippe, J.M. September 18, 2013. Lack of evidence for high fructose corn syrup as the cause of the obesity epidemic. *International Journal of Obesity*. 2013 June; 37(6): 771-773. U.S. National Library of Medicine. National Institutes of Health. Bethesda, MD 20894. Retrieved from: https://www.ncbi.nlm.nih.gov/pmc/articles/ PMC3679479/.

Lee, B. August 23, 2019. How much does insulin cost? Here's how 23 brands compare. GoodRx, Inc. Retrieved from: https://www.goodrx.com/blog/how-much-does-insulin-cost-compare-brands/.

Luhby, T. September 8, 2019. What Medicare for All would mean for the 60 million people already on Medicare. Cable News Network. Turner Broadcasting System, Inc. Atlanta, GA. Retrieved from: https://www.cnn.com/2019/09/08/politics/medicare-for-all-impact-senior-citizens/index.html.

Maddow, R., 2019. Blowout. Crown/Penguin Random House, LLC. New York, New York.

National Center for Chronic Disease Prevention and Health Promotion (US) Office on Smoking and Health. 2016. E-Cigarette Use Among Youth and Young Adults. A Report of the Surgeon General. U.S. Department of Health and Human Services, Public Health Service, Office of the Surgeon General. Rockville MD. Retrieved from: https://www.ncbi.nlm.nih.gov/books/NBK538680/pdf/Bookshelf_NBK538680.pdf.

National Minerals Information Center. U.S. Geological Survey. U.S. Department of the Interior. n.d. Salt Statistics and Information. Washington D.C. Retrieved from: https://www.usgs.gov/centers/nmic/salt-statistics-and-information.

National Shooting Sports Foundation, Inc. 2018. Firearms and Ammunition Industry Economic Impact Report 2019. Newtown CT. Retrieved from: https://d3aya7xwz8momx.cloudfront.net/wp-content/uploads/2019/02/2019-Economic-Impact.pdf.

Occupational Health and Safety Administration; U.S. Department of Labor. n.d. Toxic Industrial Chemicals (TICs) Guide. Washington D.C. Retrieved from: https://www.osha.gov/SLTC/emergencypreparedness/guides/chemical.html.

Office of the Chief Actuary. n.d. Contributions to the Social Security and Medicare Trust Funds, by program and source, 2009-2018.

Social Security Administration. Washington D.C. Retrieved from: https://www.ssa.gov/oact/STATS/table3c3.html.

Office of Public Affairs. February 1, 2011. Ohio-Based Managed Care Plan Contractor CareSource & Entities to Pay $26 million to Resolve False Claims Allegations. *Justice News*. The United States Department of Justice. Washington, D.C. Retrieved from: https://www.justice.gov/opa/pr/ohio-based-managed-care-plan-contractor-caresource-entities-pay-26-million-resolve-false.

Paul, R & Paul, K.A. 2019. The Case Against Socialism. Broadside Books/HarperCollins Publishers. New York, New York.

Ping, Z. October 10, 2019. China creates miracle in poverty reduction. People's Daily Online. *The Telegraph*. Telegraph Media Group. London, UK. Retrieved from: https://www.telegraph.co.uk/peoples-daily-online/news/poverty-reduction-in-china/.

Popken, B. October 2, 2015. America's gun business, by the numbers. CNBC. NBC News. NBC Universal. Englewood Cliffs, NJ. Retrieved from: https://www.cnbc.com/2015/10/02/americas-gun-business-by-the-numbers.html.

Régie de l'assurance maladie Québec. n.d. Social Security agreements with other countries. Gouvernement Du Québec. Québec, QC. Retrieved from: http://www.ramq.gouv.qc.ca/en/citizens/health-insurance/registration/Pages/agreements-other-countries.aspx.

Ritholtz, B. January 14. 2020. Stock ownership in the USA. The Big Picture. Ritholtz Wealth Management, LLC. Elite Cafemmedia. New York, NY. Retrieved from: https://ritholtz.com/2020/01/stock-ownership/.

Shahbandeh, M. August 9, 2019. Sugar Consumption in the U.S. 2009/10-2019/20. Statista. New York, NY. Retrieved from: https://www.statista.com/statistics/249692/us-sugar-consumption/.

Shane, Leo. September 11, 2019. Court orders VA to cover veterans' emergency room debts. *Military Times*. Sightline Media Group. Springfield, VA. Retrieved from: https://www.militarytimes.

com/news/pentagon-congress/2019/09/11/court-orders-va-t
o-cover-veterans-emergency-room-debts/.

Sohn, H. (2017, April). Racial and Ethnic Disparities in Health Insurance Coverage: Dynamics of Gaining and Losing Coverage over the Life-Course. Population Research and Policy Review. National Center for Biotechnology Information. National Library of Medicine. Retrieved from: https://www.ncbi.nlm.nih.gov/pmc/articles/PMC5370590/pdf/nihms823497.pdf.

Statista Research Department. July 22, 2019. Number of cars in the U.S. 1990-2017. Statista. New York, NY. Retrieved from: https://www.statista.com/statistics/183505/number-of-vehicles-in-the-united-states-since-1990/.

Statista Research Department. n.d. Cigars, United States. Statista. New York, NY. Retrieved from: https://www.statista.com/outlook/50030000/109/cigars/united-states.

Truth Initiative. July 19, 2018. E-cigarettes: Facts, stats, and regulations. Washington D.C. Retrieved from: https://truthinitiative.org/research-resources/emerging-tobacco-products/e-cigarettes-facts-stats-and-regulations.

U.S. Census Bureau. June 2019. Annual Estimates of the Resident Population by Sex, Age, Race and Hispanic Origin for the United States and States: April 1, 2010-July 1, 2018. American Fact Finder. U.S Department of Commerce. Washington D.C. Retrieved from: https://factfinder.census.gov/faces/tableservices/jsf/pages/productview.xhtml?src=bkmk#.

U.S. Constitution. 1789. Preamble. Applewood Books. Bedford, MA.

U.S. Department of Agriculture, Economic Research Service. October 2, 2019. Sugar and Sweeteners Yearbook Tables. Washington, D.C. Retrieved from: https://www.ers.usda.gov/data-products/sugar-and-sweeteners-yearbook-tables/sugar-and-sweeteners-yearbook-tables/#U.S.%20Sugar%20Supply%20and%20Use.

U.S. Energy Information Administration. January 2017. Fuel Oil and Kerosene Sales 2017. U.S. Department of Energy. Washington D.C. Retrieved from: https://www.eia.gov/petroleum/fueloilkerosene/pdf/foks.pdf.

U.S. Energy Information Administration. June 6, 2017. As U.S. airlines carry more passengers, jet fuel remains well below its previous peak. U.S. Department of Energy. Washington D.C. Retrieved from: https://www.eia.gov/todayinenergy/detail.php?id=31512.

U.S. Energy Information Administration. September 4, 2019. Frequency Asked Questions. How much gasoline does the United States consume? Washington D.C. Retrieved from: https://www.eia.gov/tools/faqs/faq.php?id=23&t=10.

U.S. Energy Information Administration. n.d. Petroleum & Other Liquids. Washington D.C. Retrieved from: https://www.eia.gov/dnav/pet/pet_cons_psup_dc_nus_mbbl_a.htm.

Vlastelica, R. December 22, 2017. U.S. stock trading volume hit a three-year low in 2017 amid near-absent volatility. *MarketWatch*. Dow Jones & Company. New York, NY. Retrieved from: https://www.marketwatch.com/story/us-stock-trading-volume-hit-a-three-year-low-in-2017-amid-near-absent-volatility-2017-12-21.

Wagner, I. July 17, 2019. U.S. transportation sector gasoline and distillate fuel consumption 1992-2018. Statista. New York, NY. Retrieved from: https://www.statista.com/statistics/189410/us-gasoline-and-diesel-consumption-for-highway-vehicles-since-1992/.

Wendorf, M. March 29, 2019. High Fructose Corn Syrup and the Obesity Epidemic. Interesting Engineering, Inc. San Francisco, CA. Retrieved from: https://interestingengineering.com/high-fructose-corn-syrup-and-the-obesity-epidemic.

www.ingramcontent.com/pod-product-compliance
Lightning Source LLC
Chambersburg PA
CBHW021435210526
45463CB00002B/526